Oh SH!T, I've got bowel cancer

Part One: Diagnosis and treatment diaries

Oh SH!T, I've got bowel cancer

Part One: Diagnosis and treatment diaries

DAVID BARROW

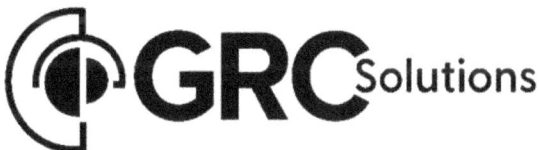

GRC Solutions
Unit 3, Clive Court
Bartholomew's Walk
Cambridgeshire Business Park
Ely, Cambridgeshire
CB7 4EA
United Kingdom
www.itgovernance.co.uk

© David Barrow 2025.

The author has asserted the rights of the author under the Copyright, Designs and Patents Act, 1988, to be identified as the author of this work.

First published in the United Kingdom in 2025 by GRC Solutions.

ISBN 978-1-78778-577-9

Cover image originally sourced from Adobe Stock, image of torso author's own.

A portion of the proceeds from every purchase of the book will be donated to Bowel Cancer UK (reg. Charity no: 1071038).

FOREWORDS

When David asked me to write the foreword to his book, I didn't hesitate for a second. David is not only a dear friend, but someone whose courage has inspired me long before this diagnosis entered his life. Like David, I too have walked through the storm of cancer. The words "you have cancer" land like a hammer blow — they stop you in your tracks, rearrange your sense of self, and force you to face questions you never imagined asking.

I first met David through the IT service management community. To be honest, I can't quite recall the moment our paths crossed — but I have no doubt it was through his tireless commitment to building community and connection. And the truth is, I'm not sure David ever cared two hoots about "service management" in the abstract. What he has always cared about is how it impacts people. That is what drew me to him, and that is what shines through in this book.

Because this isn't just a record of symptoms and treatments. It's not about processes or procedures. It's about humanity. In these pages, David shares the anger, the fear, the humour, and the gratitude that cancer drags into our lives. He reminds us that behind every diagnosis is a person, a family, and a community.

Cancer is, tragically, something that will touch half of us in our lifetime — either directly or through someone we love. Yet for all its prevalence, it remains an isolating experience.

The greatest gift we can give each other in this storm is companionship: knowing someone else has felt the same sleepless nights, the same frustration at waiting for results, the same absurdity of trying to keep life "normal" when nothing is normal at all.

David's diaries offer that gift. They remind us that while cancer can take away certainty, it cannot take away community, humour, resilience, or the will to keep moving forward.

I am proud to call David a friend, and I am honoured to introduce you to his words. May they bring you strength, comfort, and the reminder that whatever part of the journey you're on, you do not walk it alone through the pages of his book.

Katrina

About Katrina Macdermid

Katrina Macdermid hails from Australia and, through her groundbreaking framework Humanising IT™, now travels the globe helping organisations rethink the role of IT. What began as an idea has become her dream realised — training and certifying professionals worldwide and reshaping how IT is experienced by people.

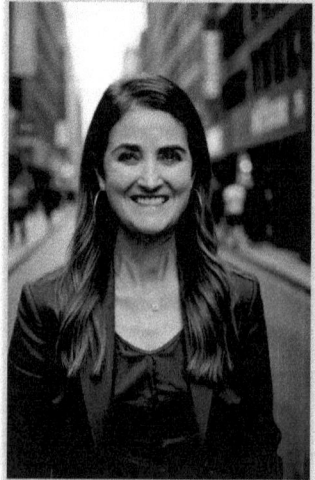

Like many of us, Katrina has faced challenges — both personal and professional. She believes it is in those moments that the right people in our lives, like David, make all the difference. His wisdom and humanity have inspired her and countless others in IT.

Outside of work, Katrina has a passion for spending time by the ocean and reading. This balance keeps her grounded as she continues her mission to make IT truly human-centred.

Having been diagnosed with cancer myself, I understand the rollercoaster of emotions that it brings to not just us, but to the people we love as well. In his book, David manages to take us on his journey, sharing his hopes and fears and at the same time providing an insight into the physical and mental challenges a diagnosis brings. Filled with fantastic resources on navigating his cancer journey and signposting charities that helped him with tips on exercise and diet, plus updates on his beloved Liverpool FC and Dorking Wanderers in the 2024/2025 season, this book is a wonderful story and resource.

The support that David receives from his team is testament to his openness and willingness to share his diagnosis, treatment plan and goals that he sets himself, which combined with his positive attitude, which is certainly tested, would make for a trophy laden season.

Everyone's cancer journey is different, though we do share similar emotions and can carry a mental burden not just for us, but for those that care for us. Through this journey, which is journalled with depth and humanity, which is still ongoing, David helps us to realise that each day is different and the peaks we aim to climb each day may lead us through a number of valleys and forests.

Whilst we may not always feel in control, this book can be a great template to help us to take charge of those things that we can, and to be advocates for our own success. The preparation that David puts into his meetings and his inquisitive nature in not only asking questions but preparing his questions in advance, remind me of my conversations with my oncology team and always having our faithful servants of how, when, where and why to understand where we are, where we are going and how to prepare.

The shock of David's diagnosis certainly doesn't affect his desire to live, which comes through in abundance, even if it does involve a few pints of Guinness, and can act as a valuable lesson in life that we don't stop living once we are told we have cancer. Life does and must go on and finding those normal activities, conversations and planning for next week, month and the future, is part of David's approach to successful survival.

I know this is the first of three books David is planning and I for one will be supporting him in his journey and looking forward to book two, three, four, five and how ever many he writes.

Hope is constant and cancer is certainly a team game.

Kevin

About Kevin Donaghy

Kevin lives with his family in the Scottish Borders. He has spent his career in IT services and IT consulting. Now living with incurable cancer, he has worked with several cancer charities in the UK, for whom he promotes causes and raises money. He has travelled the country, taking Stories of Cancer and Hope directly to the doors of various charities and people affected by cancer. His personal journey with cancer and his work with cancer charities have already featured widely in the media, with many more events planned as part of a new major publicity campaign.

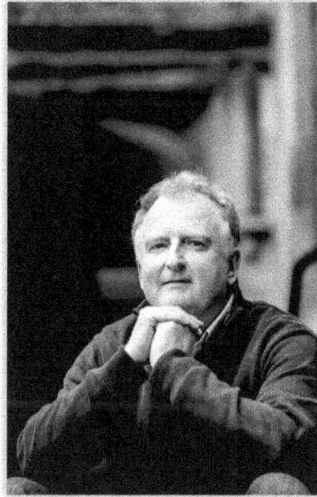

What is Sh!T, I've got bowel cancer? *Part One: Diagnosis and treatment diaries*

This book is for anyone going through cancer and wondering how to feel, what to do next, who to speak to, etc.

This book is a resource for everyone – whether you are facing cancer or supporting a loved one on their journey. The harsh reality is that one in two people will be affected by cancer at some point in their lives.[1] I sincerely hope that within these pages, you will find insights, comfort and understanding about this complex disease and its often overwhelming impact on our lives.

By shedding light on the realities of cancer, I aim to foster empathy and awareness, ultimately reminding us that we are not alone in this struggle. Each shared story and lesson learned can be a beacon of hope and support during an incredibly challenging time.

---

[1] *https://www.cancerresearchuk.org/health-professional/cancer-statistics/risk.*

ABOUT ME

I am David, also known as Dar, a 47-year-old male cancer patient who thought I had a bothersome tummy ache. That tummy ache turned out to be colorectal cancer.

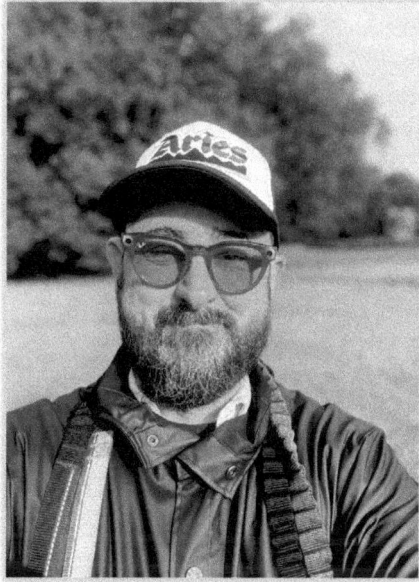

This book will document my journey from feeling poorly to going to the GP and ultimately learning I have descending colon cancer. And all the SHIT that brings with it. We begin with the diary entries that cover diagnosis, surgery and 'recovery'.

Cancer and its treatment are not a short series of events, therefore following this book I plan for there to be two further editions, all being well.

Part 2 will cover chemotherapy and Part 3 will cover whatever comes beyond medical intervention, we anticipate this being a combination of the physical and mental recovery that comes from such a life changing event.

Why did I start a diary?

This began as something deeply personal for me. I started writing diary entries as a form of journalling. At the time, I was awaiting my diagnosis, and initially, it served as a simple yet powerful tool to help me navigate my overwhelming emotions. Putting my thoughts on paper became a sanctuary where I could express my fears and hopes freely, supporting my mental health during a time when I felt completely out of control.

Writing was not just an outlet; it was therapeutic. It allowed me to process complex emotions, track my journey and gain clarity in my thoughts. At first, the diary entries served as a refuge, a space where I could make sense of the chaos surrounding me. Each entry was a step towards understanding and acceptance, helping me regain a sense of ownership in my life despite the uncertainty ahead.

As I progressed through my own experiences, I reflected on how the intimate journalling practice profoundly impacted my well-being. It helped me articulate feelings I had previously struggled to express, fostering a crucial connection to myself during that tumultuous period.

Now, as I share this diary with you, dear reader, I hope it provides support and perspective to those facing similar challenges or those supporting someone who is.

Each person experiences the news of a serious health condition differently. While this is not a comprehensive guide, it may be valuable for someone navigating their own journey. My desire to publish comes from a wish to connect with others, reminding them they are not alone and sharing resources that have significantly supported me during this whirlwind phase of my life.

THANK YOU

To my amazing wife, Emma – I could not have made it through this without you. You are the strongest person I know, and I am so grateful to have you by my side.

To my dad, Frank – your visit and love were exactly what I needed. I know you have been there for me, and I appreciate it more than you know.

To Carol and Terry – you are always there for me, and I am so proud to call you my in-laws. Jake, Matilda, Nova and Clay, you are a big part of my life and I love you all so much. Nova's flying headbutts may have hastened my trip to the doctor, but I would not trade them for anything.

To Kip – your visit made me laugh, and it hurt so bad. I will never forget your flying from Spain and back on the same day. Thank you so much for everything you have done for me.

To Tim and Shona – you revisited your experiences to help me, and I know how hard that must have been. I will always be in your debt.

To Dan, Sam, Bradley and Betsy – whether by phone or in person, I love you all so much. Thank you for being there for me during this tough time.

To Wayne, Mee Shell, Kelsie Lucas and Owen – thank you for everything you have done for me. We have shared some tough times, and I look forward to the good times ahead, including Owen getting back on those pints of Guinness.

Thank you

To Lucy – your counsel, love and humility have been so helpful during this crazy situation. Thank you so much for everything you have done for me.

To Amy, Nick, Issy, Zoe, Helen and Roger – thank you for being there for me. Each of you will always have a special place in my heart.

To Rachel, Si, Tommy, Dre, Lulu and Mark – thank you for the laughs, the visits and the league title (sorry, I could not resist).

To Suzy – I know you may think I only have reiki sessions to placate you, but that is not true. I love it, and you have helped me connect with a spirituality I only ever experienced when clubbing in the nineties.

I cannot thank everyone – you have all been so kind – but please know that your visits, messages, voice notes, emails, flowers, hampers and love mean the world to me.

You have made me cry more than once.

Thanks to the National Health Service (NHS) and cancer charities like Macmillan, Maggie's and Cancer Research UK. These organisations play a crucial role in the lives of patients fighting cancer and their families. Their unwavering support and dedication significantly improve the quality of care and emotional well-being for those affected by this life-altering illness.

The NHS provides comprehensive medical services, ensuring patients receive timely diagnoses and treatments. I went from diagnosis to surgery in just six weeks.

Their skilled healthcare professionals work hard to provide personalised care that meets each patient's unique needs, significantly improving outcomes. The NHS consistently strives to enhance cancer care, from pioneering research to innovative treatment options.

Meanwhile, cancer charities provide essential resources and support systems that go beyond medical treatment. They fund research that advances our understanding of cancer and leads to new, effective therapies. Additionally, they offer important support services, such as counselling and financial assistance, which help families cope with the challenges of cancer.

For families, this means access to emotional support, practical advice, and sometimes even social activities that help alleviate the sense of isolation that can accompany a cancer diagnosis. Organisations like Macmillan and Maggie's provide welcoming spaces where patients and their families can connect, share experiences and receive guidance from trained specialists, ensuring they are never alone.

Lastly, I want to thank Bowel Cancer UK and my publisher, IT Governance Publishing, a GRC Solutions Company, for helping me turn these diary entries into a book. I really appreciate how much Bowel Cancer UK does in research and sharing information, and I am so grateful to my publisher for taking a chance on a new book genre. Thanks to Reena, Michael, Andreas, Nicky and Kirsty for all their hard work and support on this project.

CONTENTS

Contents

THE DAY EVERYTHING CHANGED

November 2024

Before we get to my daily diary entries, providing some background and context would be handy.

I write in my diary 'in' the moment. It is a form of therapy – journalling, you may call it. Being diagnosed with cancer is awful, and I hope that if you are reading this and in a similar situation, we can get through this together.

As I write these diaries, I have no idea what the ending of this story will be. Goodness knows, I am hoping for a happy ending, but sadly, we cannot simply skip to the last page and read 'And they lived happily ever after' – in any context.

None of this stops us from hoping for a positive outcome. These diary entries will recount my journey – one I hope will be influenced by positivity, both physically and mentally.

As I said in the preface, I am a 47-year-old man who feels fit but suffers from stomach pain and cramps.

Earlier in the year (2024), as part of my ultramarathon training, I had stopped drinking alcohol for five months. When I started drinking again in the summer, I noticed discomfort in my stomach. It was not too severe but enough for me to recognise that I felt bloated, gassy and uncomfortable.

I was on holiday in Menorca in early September, and after years of not eating red meat, I suddenly craved a steak. My wife and I know the area well, so we chose the best steak restaurant, and I satisfied my craving. Within hours, I had a pain in my left side and a feeling of 'fullness' that did not leave me for an age; it was here that my stomach pains began to intensify.

On our return, I scheduled an appointment to see the doctor. Typically, that appointment was two weeks after I had made it, and I adjusted my diet a little. I dropped some more alcohol. I reduced my caffeine intake. I returned to my red-meat-free diet, drank more water, added more fruit and vegetables, and felt I was getting better, so I cancelled the appointment.

Those stomach pains returned and became more severe during a visit to Glasgow in October. They were not intense enough to stop me in my tracks, but they were noticeable while playing wrestling with my nephew. Especially after an evening of eating a Quorn-based bolognese – I was in such terrible pain that night.

So, here we were now, in early November. I realised that the pain and discomfort had returned, and I was contemplating whether I might have irritable bowel syndrome (IBS), possibly inflammatory bowel disease (IBD) or perhaps an ulcer, so I visited the doctor.

I did not think I had cancer.

When I saw the doctor, she was lovely. She asked me about my symptoms. She examined my stomach, and as she pressed on the left-hand side of my stomach, she said: "Does that hurt?"

My initial response was "no", but it shifted slightly when she released the pressure. The doctor gave me a look that, in hindsight, led me to believe this was the first time someone thought I had cancer.

She then told me I needed to do some tests.

"They will be stool samples. While I don't believe you have cancer, we need to check."

This was the first time the 'C' word was mentioned to me.

The next morning, I collected my stool samples and dropped them off on my way to a friend's birthday party in Whitstable. We had a wonderful weekend, but I experienced a lot of pain and decided not to drink.

In the end, I had a glass of delicious wine that evening and all my friends had a great time. So did I, although the pain was quite bad. Some Night Nurse medicine helped me sleep.

The results arrived on the Thursday of that following week but came in a text message. I was already having a bad day, and this compounded my feelings.

"We need to speak to you urgently about a possible cancer diagnosis."

This nearly knocked me off my chair.

I had achieved a high score for once, but in this case, it was not the high score you aim for. I had taken a FIT test. This is a 'Q'antiv faecal immunochem test' for the medical profession, but let us stick with FIT.

In this case, an acceptable score is 0 to 5. I learned that the FIT test measures blood in your stools. I've never had blood in any of my stools, not recently, not ever.

That said, I scored over 200 on that test. I've realised that some people score in the thousands, but at that moment, the thought that it could be cancer first occurred to me, and I started to worry.

In the following weeks, I was due to attend and speak at events in Manchester and Helsinki, Finland, but I cancelled them because I was on a two-week waiting list for an urgent colonoscopy.

That urgent referral meant I could be called any time in the next two weeks to make my appointment, and I did not want to drag this out any longer than was needed.

Depending on your perspective, I am either lucky or unlucky to be just minutes away from the hospital that performs colonoscopies. I informed them they could call me any time and I would be ready to schedule my appointment.

What I did not know was that (a) I would have to starve myself; and (b) take a couple of drinks that would completely empty my bowels, and I mean EMPTY my bowels.

Over the next few days, I waited for my appointment, which was finally scheduled for Sunday, 1 December 2024.

I spent that Saturday and Sunday close to the toilet. It was undignified. It was unpleasant, but ultimately, it led me to 1 December, when I had a colonoscopy that found the tumour.

Lying there on my side, I saw the ugly beast come into view, telling the person with a camera up my arse, "That doesn''t look good.""

"SHIT, I've got cancer?" I asked.

"We'll discuss it outside. Let's talk about it afterwards," he responded as he stuck a needle into it. I would later learn that this was a biopsy.

SHIT got quite real that day, and so the diary entries began.

1 DECEMBER 2024 – THE COLONOSCOPY

The day my world changed.

As the day began, I realised that the biggest inconvenience regarding the colonoscopy was being unable to eat or drink for over 24 hours and its timing, primarily because I would miss the Liverpool v Manchester City game.

Incidentally, Liverpool would go on to win 2-0, providing a strange parallel in life similar to when my mum was slowly leaving this world. In December 2019, Liverpool also sat at the top of the league. It was what kept me going during dark times. They hadn't won the league for 20 years; this was the season they finally broke that spell.

And here, in 2024, as I waited for my colonoscopy, I couldn't help but think, if Liverpool wins today's game, does this mean I'll be going through something bad in my personal life again?

The colonoscopy itself wasn't too bad. I don't like needles, but when they inserted the needle to draw my blood, it didn't bother me much, just as when they placed a cannula for sedation.

I don't remember feeling any sedation at all, and the actual procedure itself wasn't painful. It wasn't terrible. All I could feel was someone rummaging inside me.

What was awful was seeing the tumour on the screen. I know I'm no doctor, but I could tell that this wasn't right. A black mass with white fatty bits on it looming into view is something I'll never forget.

"Shit, I've got Cancer?" Reviewing these diary entries months later, I still have nightmares about this moment.

I immediately said to the man with his tube up my arse that it didn't look right. He responded, "Let's talk about it afterwards." I then felt him put some other bits and bobs inside me, and I later realised that they were taking biopsies to understand if what they had found was cancerous.

And just like that, the colonoscopy was completed in just 20 minutes. I was taken to another room where I snacked on some biscuits because I was starving and drank some terrible apple juice, all while convincing myself that what they'd found couldn't possibly be a cancerous tumour.

Unbeknown to me, they had called my wife, Emma, and said she needed to pick me up to talk with the doctor and me. I had been lying there having the colonoscopy, unaware of the worry she was experiencing, even though I knew that what I'd seen inside me wasn't right. Poor Emma was already fearing the worst.

So, Emma and I sat down, and the doctor came out. I can't recall what he said, but he mentioned that he had found a tumour that we needed to analyse.

I remember saying. "Shit, I've got Cancer?" For the second time that day.

He said it could be, but we needed to analyse it.

My next question was how I could help myself. He suggested following a low-fibre diet, which comprised the entire conversation, except for his note that receiving the results would take two to three weeks.

With that, we went home; staying with us that weekend were Emma's parents. They were waiting, and we told them that a tumour had been found, possibly the most surreal evening of my life.

I tried to escape it by watching the Liverpool game. I already knew the score. We all sat in silence for a few moments until I decided I needed to be alone and went to bed.

Believe it or not, I slept well that night. I have no idea why. Maybe it was the shock. Perhaps it was the lack of food for 36 hours because, believe me, I didn't have any dinner when I got home, even though Emma had prepared a Sunday roast. I just went to sleep and held onto my pillow, and for a little while during the night, I cried.

2 December 2024

The day after my colonoscopy, I'm still in a daze, trying to process the news. A tumour – how could this happen to me? Since turning 40, I've wanted to live a healthy life and treat my body well. Why now?

Emma is supportive, telling me we'll get through this together. But I'm terrified of the future, the unknown, and confronting my mortality. The uncertainty of what lies ahead is paralysing. I'm overwhelmed by a blend of despair, anger and numbness. When I close my eyes, all I can see is the image of that alien growth marring my insides. I've never felt so betrayed by my own body.

> **Note: I hope that sharing these emotions helps you feel connected and less alone in your struggles if you are going through something similar.**

Today, I receive a phone call and I'm informed that I need a CT scan, which involves another cannula and a set of needles. Great.

> **How can I get through this limbo while waiting for the test results? I alternate between despair, anger, and numbness.**

Emma keeps telling me to take it one day at a time and stay positive. However, when I'm alone, I find myself desperate to cry, yet unable to. I'm not ready for this fight; I don't know if I have the strength for what's to come. Nonetheless,

I must try for Emma and for the life we've built together. Her support, along with the support of my loved ones, is what keeps me going. I'm grateful for their love and understanding, and I hope you also have such a strong support system in your life.

My mind continually wanders; I always thought I had more time – time to do everything I've put off – travel the world again, make more pottery, complete Gran Turismo 7, and tell my loved ones what they mean to me.

My time feels finite, but I'm determined not to waste what is left.

Starting today, I will live with purpose, gratitude and love. Although this tumour may have grown inside me, it does not define me. I define myself by how I choose to live. I refuse to let this illness dictate my life. I will embrace each day with intention, making the most of every moment.

3 December 2024

It's just another working day. I feel numb. Nothing seems important, and the world is spinning off its axis around me. I move onto the bed and sleep. That positivity I held yesterday has disappeared, and my emotions are a rollercoaster. What once felt important now feels unimportant, and I'm unable to function properly.

4 December 2024

CT Scan Day. Two attempts to get the cannula in and the joy of drinking one litre of water in the hour before a procedure where they say that I might feel like I'm wetting myself – while inside a machine with my hands above my head. I don't piss myself, but I feel like I do.

I laugh to myself at how surreal things are right now.

Liverpool draws 3-3 with Newcastle. Mo Salah wants that new contract; give that man his contract!

5 December 2024

I've told my client what's going on; she's amazing. Informing those who need to know is liberating. My world is returning to an even keel, and I'm regaining some control. My client is also a reiki master – her name is Suzy. Suzy is an exceptional human, and before we sign off, she offers me remote reiki that evening. I have no idea how it works, but it's fucking brilliant, truly brilliant.

We also discuss my water intake. I'm pleased to say that I drink two litres daily, but during this chat, we also touch on the fact that I only drink sparkling water. As soon as I mention it, Suzy and I both think and say the same thing:

"Could the sparkling water be unhelpful for bloating?"

It's so obvious as I write, so I cut out sparkling water, and the difference is huge; I feel tons better within a day. I've lost no weight, but my bloating has gone and my favourite jeans fit within days. Thank you, Suzy!

6 December 2024

I woke up feeling resolved. Last night, I had remote reiki, during which I visualised myself as calm, purposeful and committed to controlling this tumour.

Those first few seconds of waking up are normal, but how you manage that immediate smack in the face informs your day. Today, the pain in my side, which, TBH, could all be in my mind, is nagging at me. I go to the gym with Emma.

I ran 5 km in Delft in November, but it felt so hard back then, a real struggle and my lungs couldn't handle it that day. Looking back and following the CT scan, I begin to wonder if this tumour has spread to my lungs. The worst fears occupy my mind as I step onto the machine.

I base this on the fact that I ran 50 km earlier this year, which was tough, but this 5 km today feels mentally tougher. I can usually run 5 km in 23 minutes, but I'll be happy if I put in a 30-minute effort today.

I get on the machine and set it to 5 km at a 10 km/hour pace; at this pace, I'll complete the distance in 30 minutes. Those first steps feel great. Five minutes in, I increase to 10.5 km/hour, then 11 km/hour at 12 minutes. I finish my 5 km in 27 minutes with loads left in the tank.

Fuck you, tumour!

7 December 2024

Everton v Liverpool has been postponed, and I've lost the two hours I had set aside to immerse myself. My dad and his wife are staying with us, and it's a bloody awful day weather-wise. A trip to a wine estate and a country pub for a fish-finger sandwich, blackcurrant and soda doesn't make up for this.

However, we enjoy a meal in the evening, and I even have two pints of Guinness – a rare treat nowadays. I had cut down on alcohol before and felt it was the right thing to do; however, the temptation to turn two into twenty is strong.

I head to bed tonight, realising that life continues; we must adapt to a new normal.

8 December 2024

My dad and Maggie leave us to head home and back to the north. I've no doubt I'll survive this episode, but it feels strange that I probably won't see Dad before I start my treatment plan. Maybe I'll be sliced open or bald when we meet again. I'll certainly have more scars, physically and mentally.

I settle down and watch the final F1 race of the season. It's another dull race, but it distracts me for a bit. I've never truly been one to seek distractions, but I suppose that needs to change now.

9 December 2024

Over the weekend, I felt overwhelmed by negative thoughts. During moments of anxiety, I found myself searching for information about my tumour and the pain in my side, which only made me feel more irrational. I've been experiencing pain on my left side, a discomfort that began after my colonoscopy. I anxiously await my test results, and my thoughts keep swinging between optimism and fear. I know that Google is the enemy in this situation, but I can't help myself.

Suppose you're reading this and find yourself in a similar situation. In that case, I want to highlight two excellent sites

I find far better than Google – exploring these alleviated some of my concerns and helped calm my scattered thoughts.

- Bowel Cancer UK: *https://www.bowelcanceruk.org.uk/*.
- Macmillan Cancer Support:
  https://www.macmillan.org.uk/.

Both have forums where people share the same emotions you are feeling or have felt.

Please go there, not to Google.

These forums also suggested that I stay in touch with the nurses on the multi-disciplinary teams (MDTs), as they often have insight into what's happening with each case. I called the nurses and was informed that I might be on the agenda for tomorrow's meeting; they advised me to call back tomorrow afternoon to see if I could learn more. I instantly feel empowered, and while I try not to get carried away, I now feel I understand more about their process, which is helpful.

10 December 2024

We're now ten days post-colonoscopy, and I hope to get my results today.

Last night, I slept for over eight hours; one thing I've tried to do amid all this is sleep well. My sleep is an escape, but it also heals me.

Emma and I go to the gym again. This time, I cover 5.68 km in 30 minutes. Ironically, I signed up for a half-marathon in April to support my father-in-law's prostate cancer diagnosis, and I now plan to go through with it, no matter what.

I need to check if this is achievable.

At 12:30 pm, I give in and call the colorectal unit at East Surrey Hospital. I speak with a kind nurse named Nicky, who explains everything to me.

In short.

I have cancer.

I need bowel surgery.

It's a 'curative' procedure.

My first feeling is one of relief. I have a cyst on one of my kidneys that requires an MRI, but in short, they're not concerned about it.

The results

On a scale of 1 to 10, where 1 is 'terminal' and 10 is 'perfectly healthy', I would estimate my condition at a 6. I anticipated surgery, and now I need to prepare for it.

I never thought I'd be so over the moon about having my insides torn apart. Now, I can get to grips with things.

Within hours, I've booked my MRI scan, my surgeon meeting and my surgery.

The surgery is booked for 13 January 2025. My wife Emma's birthday.

We share with friends and family, and most are shocked to learn that we feel relieved, but that's the reality. Considering the worst-case scenario, this feels like a positive outcome. With any luck, this cancer will be removed in five weeks' time.

Now for my next challenge: work. I'm self-employed, and my current engagement is nearing its end. How the fuck do I find a job in this depressed market when I face a potential three-month recovery and possibly chemotherapy to come? As one problem disappears, another arises.

I celebrate with chocolate. Just four weeks ago, the 'old' me would've opted for a Guinness or five. But not now. I want to be in the best shape for this surgery. Not that chocolate is a healthy food, but you get me!

That night, Liverpool edges past Girona 1-0. Once again, they distract me from my worries, just as they did when Mum died five years ago.

5 YEARS AGO

16 December 2019

After a long few years of alcohol abuse, depression and self-abuse, my poor mum passed away just a few hours after I had left her the night before.

She had been in and out of the ICU for two years, losing the use of her legs and never finding the willpower to regain that ability. This, among all her behaviours, angered me the most. She didn't give herself the best chance for a successful recovery and rehabilitation, and it boiled inside me.

Upon her death, my overriding emotion was relief – a feeling I find so heartless to express. After several years, I no longer have to rush for emergencies. Riding my motorbike up and down the motorways had worried me and my wife, Emma; my mind was often preoccupied with what I might find upon arrival rather than fully focused on the road.

Our holidays were often disrupted by another issue with Mum, any arrangements felt more stressful rather than a pleasure.

I stood in the hospital room that day, looking down at my mother's still body. I was with my aunts, holding Mum's hand, and it was the worst thing I've ever done – writing this is awful, but she felt so cold, so DEAD. Nowadays, I genuinely cannot pick up our dog's cold poo, as it gives me the same feeling.

5 years ago

As I released her hand, a wave of relief washed over me, quickly followed by a swell of guilt. She had not been an easy woman to care for, especially in those last few years as her health declined. But she was still my mother. And now she was gone.

I reflected on all the times I had rushed to her side, never knowing what condition I would find her in. The falls, the episodes with alcohol, the caregivers being mistreated by her and accused of theft. I thought about my 90-year-old grandmother, who had to endure this as well. My aunties were incredible; they lived nearby and did everything they could, but I reminded myself that she was my responsibility.

Now that the burden had been lifted, the freedom felt strange. There were no more late-night calls to worry about and no more rearranging plans – just stillness and silence.

I headed back home and suddenly felt very alone. What kind of son was I to be so relieved at her passing? She had tried her best in her way. Now, we would both have to make peace with a complicated past. That night, I just wanted to be with my wife, Emma, and my dog, Norris. We went for a drink to toast Mum. We have a picture of that night. I'm smiling in the picture, but I was dying inside.

As I went to sleep that night, I tossed and turned. At about 3 am, I decided to give myself some closure. "Goodbye, Mum," I whispered. "I hope you find some peace." I then buried my head in the pillow.

January 2020

The funeral.

5 years ago

I sat alone in the funeral home, staring at the simple wooden casket that held my mother's body. A sense of numbness had taken hold, making it hard to process the mix of emotions swirling inside me. Relief, anger, regret and sadness all blended into a dull ache in my chest.

Now, here I sat, reflecting on my last hospital visit in the early hours before she died; I chose to drive home at 2 am since I had work the next day. Yet here I was, wishing I had been gentler in those final hours. Wishing I had embraced her fragile frame and told her I loved her despite our strained relationship. But the guilt and the 'what if's were pointless now. She was gone.

I wondered if she had sensed that the end was near and if that was why she clutched my hand a little as I left. I realised then that she had been reaching out quietly while I recoiled.

Tears stung my eyes as regret washed over me. Despite the anger, I hoped she knew that a little boy still loved his mummy. I wished she could forgive me for not understanding until it was too late.

That night, the night of the funeral, we drove home, followed by friends. For them, this was 100 miles further from home than necessary. We went for pints and curry; I'll never forget their support.

Why the flashback?

They say that grief can affect you in many ways; for me, it manifested as bitterness and anger, and I truly wonder if this darkness led to the tumour. I'm not blaming Mum;

instead, I'm blaming myself for not addressing my emotions – this diary is my effort to avoid repeating that mistake.

If only I had handled the grief differently. If only I had allowed someone in to help me through it instead of pushing my emotions away. There are so many 'if only's' now, but none of them matter any more. The only thing I can do is figure out how to confront this tumour and let go of the anger before it's too late.

This diary marks the beginning; it's time to start healing both body and spirit.

The road ahead will be difficult, but I will not walk it alone. I will not follow my mother's lead; a date for surgery gives me something to prepare for and to 'train' my body and mind for.

Tumour, I'm coming for you.

11 December 2024

My last day of work before Christmas is bittersweet since I'm uncertain when I can work again for a prolonged period. My operation is scheduled for 13 January 2025. Between now and then, I can only work for five days in January, so Emma and I will have just five days of money to live on.

Are we facing a health and financial crisis?

This is likely to be my last day working for a while, perhaps even forever, and that realisation weighs heavily on me. My risky operation is just a few weeks away. After that, my recovery will be long and uncertain.

Sighing, I turn off my computer and look around my home office. I've enjoyed working with this client, and I appreciate the meaningful tasks and the supportive colleagues. However, illness and its heavy financial burden now threaten not only my health but also our economic stability.

In my own research, I've found that a report commissioned by Digestive Cancers Europe indicates that bowel cancer costs the UK economy £1.74 billion annually. This figure includes indirect expenses, such as lost income and unpaid care from friends and relatives. Such financial burdens significantly impact patients and caregivers, intensifying the economic strain of a diagnosis.

Source: *https://www.bowelcanceruk.org.uk/news-and-blogs/news/bowel-cancer-costs-the-uk-%C2%A31.74-billion-a-year/*.

Bowel Cancer UK also offers valuable advice about finances on their web pages; I find this very useful to refer to: *https://www.bowelcanceruk.org.uk/how-we-can-help/family-friends-carers-support/money/*.

I also speak to my local Macmillan centre, which offers me assistance via Citizens Advice, something I act upon straight away.

Citizens Advice not only advise me on handling my self-employed income but also asks me if I have any other income and/or insurance policies to speak of. This chat reminds me to speak to my financial advisor.

Through these conversations, I've discovered I'm not alone.

If I were very frugal, my savings might cover a few months of expenses after the surgery. But beyond that, we face an uncertain future on both medical and monetary fronts. This is a stressful double blow requiring courage, which I'm not sure I possess.

But I know others face even worse diagnoses and prognoses. I hope that science and some holiday spirit will see me through. This Christmas may be bittersweet, but it'll be one I won't forget

12 December 2024

I partner with Dorking Wanderers FC, a local non-league football team through my business. As a shareholder, I see how my investment and that of others are being developed and are supporting the local community.

We have a great morning with the club, learning about their plans and participating in a penalty shoot-out. I win a competition taking penalties against the first team goalie; 'win' – I'm the last out with two scored. I'll take it.

This is the first time in several weeks that I've managed to forget there's something wrong with me, and it's the first time since I learned I had cancer that I've forgotten about my diagnosis.

It's the first time the world has felt normal since I first said "Shit – I've got bowel cancer" .

It's the first time I've felt like myself since then to and I believe it's the first time I've genuinely laughed or smiled since that day. While that upsets me, it's also a wonderful day filled with laughter, new ideas, getting to know people, and reflecting on what I want to do with my business once I overcome this challenge. One thing I've realised since feeling unwell is that the world I work in – a world where I've had some success, where I'm recognised and where I have global communities that look up to me – no longer feels important; it seems irrelevant to me right now. So, I need to contemplate what I want to pursue once I'm better, but I also have to consider what I need to do to pay the bills, which is weighing on my mind.

13 December 2024

Today is Friday, typically a joyful day and the start of everyone's weekend. It would usually mark the end of the working week, but for me, it's just another scan.

Before the MRI scan, this scan will cover several things, including looking at the cyst on my kidney, Emma and I go shopping and buy some crystals that my reiki master, Suzy, recommended I get. Honestly, I'm not sure if carrying a few stones in my pockets will help, but I'm open to trying anything now. My appointment is at 2:30 pm.

We leave at 1:30 pm and find the MRI scanning area upon our arrival at 1:45. They're running late, and I'm informed that I will need another injection so that a dye can be injected into my body. These things used to bother me, but now they're just routine needles that don't affect me. The MRI lasts 30 minutes. It's not especially terrible, but it's not exactly good either.

When I enter the machine, they ask me to breathe in and out according to its commands. Halfway through, it stops telling me when to breathe in, so I'm exhaling, trying to hold my breath for 20 seconds, and feeling like I'm turning purple.

They offer to play some music on the machine, but all they can provide is Christmas music, which is the last thing I want to hear right now. Before I know it, it's all over, and we head home.

As this treatment has progressed, I've become anxious. Although these scans may only contain good news, this anxiety isn't unusual for patients; it even has a name – **Scanxiety.**

As part of my process, I've sought out more information on what is new for me. I hope you'll find this helpful too:

- *https://www.bowelcanceruk.org.uk/news-and-blogs/this-is-bowel-cancer-blog/bowel-cancer-tests-surveillance-and-scan-anxiety/.*

In other, brighter news, tonight was a wonderful evening. Emma's friends – people I've known almost as long as I've known Emma, a solid 27 years – have gathered from different parts of the country to check on me and help take my mind off things.

Their kindness was beautiful, and I will never forget it. So, if you're reading this, thank you; it means the world to me.

14 December 2024

Emma and her friends went to watch *The Snowman* in Guildford. They all wanted to come to see me and help out; it's so lovely of them. Our friend Amy, who learned about my cancer yesterday, drove down at 6 am to see me. Wow, thank you!

They're all incredible women, and I want to publicly thank them for coming to me in my time of need.

Emma's friends are my friends.

This morning, I went to the gym and ran 5 km in 25 minutes. I've found that going for a run boosts my mood.

While the girls were out, I cleaned the house, wrote a bit in this diary and my other books, and organised myself as an Amazon author. I plan to publish this diary when I know what the future holds, so if you're reading this now, it means something happened. Let's hope it's positive.

I watched Liverpool as always. After the game, I wanted to go for a pint, and bless the girls, they decided they would like that too. When they returned home, we went for happy hour at our local village pub, which has roaring fires at this time of year and Guinness to die for. Those pints of Guinness felt great – we just sat chatting, drinking Guinness, eating bar snacks and enjoying a nice evening.

Nothing special, nothing great, just good.

Thanks, girls.

15 December 2024

Emma's friends left today. It's Sunday, and my mood is dark. I don't know what's changed, but I don't feel like myself. Even though my last conversation with the nurse was that we would be doing curative surgery, I still feel like something could go wrong. What does the MRI show? Is it something they didn't pick up before?

What if I have testicular cancer because I felt pain there after running yesterday? What if it's in my hip? I also have pain there.

What if, what if, what if?

We experience worries about our health – those thoughts that sneak into our minds, embed themselves and circulate. I've been trying to maintain a positive outlook regarding this situation, but that doesn't mean one can't sometimes dwell on the negative.

Maybe it's because I had a few pints last night. As I enjoyed my Guinness, I felt relaxed. The world seemed normal. I wasn't thinking about cancer or dying, or being cut open in operations. I was thinking that it was just a regular Saturday night. I didn't get drunk. I didn't go wild. I had a few pints, and everything felt normal.

However, today, when I woke up, everything felt different. I was scared. I felt alone even though I wasn't. I wondered how I was going to fight this.

16 December 2024

I'm not sure there's anything like a normal Monday any more, but it felt like a normal Monday today.

Emma and I planned to go to the gym but couldn't be bothered. Instead, we took the dogs (we now have two, with Frank joining us last year), for a walk and relaxed. We then started preparing the house for Christmas. Friends and family are coming over, and people will drop in and out for the holiday. We told them we wanted to keep this up simply because I need the distractions.

And on this day, even though I'm writing it on the day, I can't recall anything that sticks out.

Yes, I was thinking about cancer, worrying about money and our financial security, and wondering whether I would still be here next year, but now it was in dispatches rather than me dwelling on it. While waiting for the test results, I went out and bought a PlayStation 5; it's the kind of thing I do to distract myself. In the afternoon, I played Gran Turismo to keep myself occupied.

17 December 2024

Today, I woke up still worried about the cancer and am now concerned about my appointment with the surgeon in the coming days.

I have so many thoughts filling my mind that I must purge them. Believe it or not, not having any work at the moment is genuinely a pain in the arse. Not only am I concerned about our financial security, but I also can't relax. I can't enjoy my time off, which is frustrating at this time of year. Therefore, I decided to prepare myself for some work as a self-employed individual to get ready for next year. This means I can organise my books, prepare my wife's tax return, and tackle our bills to manage those annoying life chores that persist when you're worried about dying from cancer.

That said, I managed to let go of some of those worries. I went for another run today. This time, I decided to train for the half-marathon that I'm doing in April.

I have no idea if I'll make the start line for that half-marathon, but my plan has always been to run it in two hours or less. So today, I aimed to run for an hour at a pace that would allow me to finish the half-marathon in two hours or less, and that's exactly what I did. I covered 10.6 km in 55 minutes, and as I did so, I started shaming my tumour.

As I ran on that machine, I told the tumour it wouldn't win. I stated it wouldn't stop me, and I developed a new resolve to ensure that when I have the chance, I will run that half-marathon. I will complete it in under two hours and continue to fight this bastard.

18 December 2024

Tomorrow is my outpatient appointment for colorectal surgery, and I'm not sure what it entails. I believe it means we'll discuss my cancer, my surgery, and whether I'll need chemotherapy once the surgery is finished.

Emma and I are making a list of questions using the notes app on my phone; even talking to one another about my cancer diagnosis is overwhelming. It still feels like this is happening to someone else.

Tonight, Liverpool played Southampton away in the League Cup. They won 1-2 and advanced to the semi-finals. Thanks, Redmen, for another great two hours of distraction.

IT'S CHRISTMAS

19 December 2024

Today was the day we met the surgeon. First, I want to express how grateful I am for the NHS. It's incredible to think that just a few weeks ago, we had no idea what was happening, and today we found ourselves sitting in front of a surgeon discussing the surgery scheduled for 13 January next year.

When we sat down, we had a list of questions. Fortunately for me, the surgeon explained what he would do and answered the vast majority of our questions as he went along. They know this information so well.

This might come off as big-headed, but it felt like I was looking at him and comparing him to myself in my field of work, where I'm regarded as a 'thought leader'. I noticed he was practised, familiar with multiple scenarios, and very aware of my presence. It felt personal. I had also checked his public profile, which was helpful; sensing his confidence was reassuring.

He is going to remove the lower left part of my bowel. If all goes well, that's all they'll take out, but if getting in there is awkward or difficult, they'll need to remove more of my bowel, maybe all of it. The surgeon spoke about this as though it were something he normally does, such as eating breakfast or waking up in the morning.

This reassured me that I would be in the right hands when I was put under.

I believe we got through most of that list of questions, but as soon as I left, I realised there was one more: just how big is my tumour?

This is where having someone else helps. Emma picked up on this and reminded me that the surgeon mentioned the camera they put inside me couldn't even get past the tumour, which shows it must be quite large.

If you are in this situation, I recommend taking someone with you.

You can read more about this here:

- *https://patient.info/news-and-features/what-not-to-say-to-someone-with-cancer.*

I asked how I could help myself, and he said I'm to maintain a low-fibre diet, but he also said not to eat or drink like a monk and get myself through to 13 January so they can cut this bastard out.

Here are the questions we asked, along with the answers:

- *How long will the surgery take?* **A – 5 hours!**
- *What type of surgery is it?* **A – They're aiming for keyhole surgery but may need to revert to open surgery.**
- *How long will I be in hospital for?* **A – 4–10 days.**
- *Can I do anything to help myself before surgery?* **A – Eat a low-fibre diet, exercise, and enjoy Christmas.**
- *Is this a curative surgery?* **A – That's the plan.**

- *What happens in the days/weeks/months after?* **A** – I will undergo an Enhanced Recovery plan, and my tumour will be analysed alongside some healthy tissue to see if I need any further treatment.
- *Am I too ambitious to plan to run a half-marathon in April, 83 days post-surgery?* **A** – Far too ambitious (gutted). Try a parkrun instead.
- *When can I walk our strong dogs again?* **A** – 6 weeks.
- *What should I eat and drink afterwards?* **A** – Soft food for a few days; slowly reintroduce fibre and fruit/veg/nuts.
- *Will I be free from cancer post-surgery?* **A** – I will need the test results.
- *Do I need chemo?* **A** – I will need the test results.
- *Do I need radiation?* **A** – Not applicable for this cancer.
- *What is the likelihood it'll come back?* **A** – There's a chance. I'll be on an observation programme for five years.
- *What should I bring to the hospital?* **A** – myself; toiletries; underwear; baggy, comfy clothes; PJs; headphones; and a long charger lead.
- *Will I need a stoma?* **A** – We'll only know as we operate. You will be prepared for one!
- *Will he die?* **Emma's question to the surgeon. A** – We plan for him to live for many years afterwards.

To celebrate, Emma and I went to our local bar for a few drinks. This seemed like the best way to deal with the bad news. Now, all we have to do is make it to 13 January.

The surgeon told me that I couldn't run the half-marathon 83 days after the surgery, but he mentioned that I could keep training before then, and he hopes I can run a 5 km parkrun within that period. So, that's what I'm now going to aim for:

Parkrun, I'm on my way.

We headed home, and I feel relieved knowing what lies ahead, including the uncertainties. Bring it on.

20 December 2024

Today is supposed to be the last working Friday before Christmas, but for me, it's the day after learning about my surgery.

I wake up with mixed emotions because I should be happy that, in an ideal world, they're going to remove this cancer and that it'll be gone. However, the problem is that I looked at the Internet last night. I researched how much pain people endure when they have these operations, as well as how little they may suffer, but I focused on the negative.

We go shopping since we're having everyone over for Christmas; we need food and drinks. We also take a drive, if only to clear our heads. It's an ordinary day, but sometimes it's just what you need to feel better and think clearly.

21 December 2024

Today is a good day. We drive to Bracknell to visit one of my friends, who has come down from Manchester with his kids to go to LaplandUK. We catch up, go to the park, push the kids on the swings, enjoy a nice brunch, and discuss cancer. It's comforting to talk to people who understand me and recognise that I'm processing it, yet also keep me grounded, provide humour and help me forget about it; it's a pleasant day out.

It's a good drive, and on the way home, I buy the Christmas booze, even though I won't enjoy it too much this year.

22 December 2024

Today, I once again wake up feeling anxious; anxiety is something I've never experienced in my life before. I've always been quite confident and outspoken in my self-belief, but today, I'm anxious. I'm worried, I'm scared, and this is the first period of my life where this has happened to me.

Emma and I take the dogs for a lovely long walk, yet all I can think about is whether this might be the last time or one of the last times I take the dogs for a walk, even though I know that's not the case.

We go to Marks & Spencer. Wow, what a highlight! It's a highlight because I'm self-employed, which allows me to gift Emma and me director vouchers to spend anywhere we want – in this case, M&S. Doing so means we get a lot of food for free, and it's good fun.

We get to choose anything we want from the shelves. It's like a supermarket sweep for the finest treats, the best preserves, and all the delightful bits and bobs for Christmas. This morning, we indulged in a middle-class activity and visited a quaint market near our home. I bought some olives and pickled onions, and believe it or not, I managed to spend £14 on these items. That will serve me right for getting free food at M&S!

Even better today, the mighty Liverpool FC showed us that it's beginning to feel a SLOT-like Christmas as they put six goals past Tottenham Hotspur and cemented their position at the top of the Premier League. For me, this is a wonderful distraction. It's a way to forget what's going on in life and to want to get to Liverpool.

23 December 2024

I wake up and decide to go for a run at the gym. When I arrive at the gym, in a strange twist of fate, I see the lady who was at the reception during my colonoscopy. We've often encountered each other at the gym, but I only realised she worked at the hospital after my appointment.

She is incredibly lovely. She introduces herself as Wendy and asks me how I'm doing and how things had gone, so I share the results with her. Talking to her is quite encouraging.

It turns out she knows the surgeon operating on me. She says the man works miracles and asserts that I'm in great hands. That little pep talk is uplifting. We both finish our runs and wish each other a Merry Christmas, and I feel a bit happier than before getting on the treadmill.

Today is the day everyone begins to arrive at our house, starting with my mother-in-law and father-in-law, Carol and Terry.

They join us for a street party that our road hosts yearly, which is again wonderful. It's nice to see everyone. We have new neighbours, and it's great to welcome them to the street party. We inform a couple of the neighbours about what's happening because Emma will need assistance. She's going to need help walking the dogs and with general lifting and tasks like that, which I can't do for about six weeks after the operation. It's hard to explain to people what's going on, but it's the right thing to do. They can help us because they're good people, and good people like to assist their neighbours; one day, I know I'll be able to return the favour.

The street part is really fun. I have a couple of drinks and eat some carrots since everything else is red meat, and red meat isn't good for cancer. Ultimately, I have a great time.

24 December 2024

Christmas Eve is typically my favourite day of the year, and I'm resolute that this day will be no exception. Emma goes to a pantomime with her whole family while I stay back at the house to wrap her stocking fillers.

This family has stockings, main presents and tree presents. Even after 20-some years in the family, I still don't understand how it works. I wrap things up and decide what goes where on the day.

I have my own tradition: watching Bourne films while wrapping presents. They're long, but I know them so well that I don't need to watch them. I find it relaxing, and today, I feel quite calm.

After the pantomime, my family comes over, and my uncle, cousin and I go to the pub for a drink. It's amazing how nice it feels to do something I used to do often but now do rarely.

It's a familiarity. I'm not an alcoholic by any means. I enjoy going to the pub. I want to chat with people and embrace the world around me, which helps me forget what's happening inside.

However, I'm rudely reminded of what's happening inside me when we go for a curry later that evening, which has also become a tradition. I must think carefully about which dish to order, as I've discovered that spices, which are one of my favourite things, don't react well with my tumour. So, I opt for a chicken shashlik and a lentil dish. It's still delicious, but it's not quite what I would've chosen before.

25 December 2024

Christmas Day. This is not a Christmas like those I've experienced before. I'm not excited about Christmas; indeed, my first thought when I wake up is, "Shit, I've got cancer and I have to undergo an operation to carve it out in a few weeks."

It's strange waking up and feeling normal for just a few seconds, only to realise that there's something inside of you that's trying to infect and kill you. Now, I'm fairly realistic and understand that my cancer isn't doing that yet, but I know I have to be cut open to remove the bugger, which presents a whole new set of problems to consider.

However, it's Christmas, and my wife, Emma, and I have a small tradition of lying in bed and exchanging stockings before anyone else can see us. We also have stockings for our dogs, Norris and Frank. These stockings are enjoyable and never too serious; they're simply gifts we appreciate. They allow us to spend some peaceful time before the madness descends.

However, today will be quite a quiet day. Only Emma's parents will be with us, as Emma's brother Jake, his partner Matilda and their two children, Nova and Clay, will join us tomorrow.

Today is quite relaxed. We take it easy in the morning, have breakfast and walk the dogs. Then, from 12–2 pm, we meet friends at our local pub. After that, we return home to unwind on the sofa and watch the finale of *Gavin and Stacey* on the BBC.

Overall, it's a quiet day, but slightly different from usual because I monitor what I eat and drink. I'm ensuring I have an alcoholic drink, but not too many. I spend most of the day drinking flavoured water and staying hydrated, which is quite good. Not going to bed feeling massively bloated is pretty cool.

Boxing Day – 26 December 2024

Today is the day we welcome more family members. We spend the morning cleaning the house, preparing for it to get dirty again.

My brother-in-law, his partner and their two boys are joining us today. Nova is four years old, bursting with energy, and Clay is just five months old. He's the most smiley, adorable little boy you could ever meet.

Having everyone around, especially the two boys, is a delightful distraction from what's happening in the world and my stomach. It's truly enjoyable to play with the boys, hold them and see them at this wonderful time of year for them.

This evening, we have fish chowder, which I'd been looking forward to because I can eat copious amounts without worrying too much about its fibre content – fibre is, in my case, the enemy. One upside of this diet is that I no longer feel bloated. I also no longer feel pain, strangely. I no longer feel as if I've got cancer, even though that's exactly what I have.

27 December 2024

Today is our family's main Christmas Day; I will head to the gym before we begin.

New Year, new me?

I run 6 km, and I do so really well; it's me telling cancer to fuck off and leave me alone, and even though it won't do that, I feel like I get one up on it whenever I go for a run and whenever I exert myself to the point where I feel like I'm doing something that makes me feel stronger and better and more prepared for my surgery.

This Boxing Day is not without drama. After going out for a drink, we find that one of the dogs (perhaps both) has stolen and eaten all our pigs in blankets, including the cocktail sticks holding them together.

We're unsure which dog ate them, but now we must keep an eye on both to ensure they're OK. I call the vet because, at the moment, I'm in a heightened state of worry, and the vet tells me we have a couple of choices. One is to bring them in and find out which one has cocktail sticks inside them. The other is to feed them lots and lots of food, which will pack out the cocktail sticks and prevent the dogs from hurting themselves.

One of our dogs loves food, so this is an absolute dream for him. I spend most of the afternoon feeding the dogs far too much while also indulging the humans a bit too much. We have a great Christmas dinner; for my part, I take it easy on the sprouts, which is a shame since I genuinely like them.

Everybody apart from me gets slightly drunk, and we have a nice day, but for me, it still feels like something is missing, or should I say something extra is inside me? The cancer inside of me continues to capture my mind, and it's now only a couple of weeks until that bugger is removed from me.

In other news, I receive a phone call from the hospital. I had missed two previous calls. The purpose of the call is to arrange my pre-assessment for surgery and to inform me when I need to be available for surgery.

My pre-assessment will be on 6 January. I'm also looking forward to meeting an Enhanced Recovery Nurse. On 13 January, when I have my operation, I need to be at the hospital by 7 am. This isn't a big deal, as the hospital is only five minutes away, but 13 January is my wife's birthday, so it seems we won't have much time together that day.

28 December 2024

Can you believe that we're now on Christmas Day number three? Today, we're off to see family elsewhere.

I don't feel like doing this today, not because I dislike them. Quite the opposite – they're great. Some days, I don't know what mood I'll wake up in, and after yesterday's fiasco with the dogs eating the pigs in blankets, I spent the night worrying that one of them might die. As a result, I'm knackered.

It's strange how death lingers in the mind when there's something inside you that essentially exists to harm you. Again, this is just me being a glass-half-empty person.

Fortunately, I spent the time I couldn't sleep last night reading *The Source*, which teaches me how to think positively. It still works for me today when I wake up and my mind tries to reset to a default of angst and worry.

- *https://www.taraswart.com/the-source/*.

What a wonderful day we have! Many children and adults have fun, and there's lots of food, including an incredible lasagne from my Italian cousin.

All in all, it's a great day. What's lovely is that as I leave, they say they're thinking about me and will send me positive vibes on 13 January.

Thank you, everybody, for making my day lovely. You didn't even know you were doing it, but you did.

29 December 2024

Today is the day our first Christmas guests leave. It's sad to say goodbye, not because I genuinely think it's the last time I'll ever see them. Still, I know it's the last time I'll see them before I go for this operation and find out if I need chemotherapy. I'm vain, and I wonder if it's the last time I'll see them with my hair.

It's crazy how strange things go through your mind. It also means that we're a step closer to reality, a step closer to confronting the fact that in just a couple of weeks, I'm going to have my stomach sliced open and my cancer removed.

30 December 2024

The day begins with another run; once again, I tell cancer to fuck off repeatedly as I run 7 km in under 35 minutes. I know I'm probably pushing myself too hard, but it feels good.

It feels great!

Today, Emma's parents are leaving us to go back home.

So far, in these diaries, I've hardly mentioned that Emma's dad is also battling cancer. He has prostate cancer, which is at stage two, and he's beginning radiotherapy treatment tomorrow – on New Year's Eve. I feel for him; what a way to spend New Year.

I glance at Emma's dad and applaud him for managing everything. He, like me, thinks waiting for news and test results is the worst part.

I think that anyone reading this who is waiting to find out if they have cancer, or waiting for anything else, should know that the waiting is the hardest part. Once you know you have a plan and a way to deal with it, things begin to get easier, but they never become easy.

Bowel Cancer UK has some great resources that offer tips on this time, which I find especially useful:

* *https://www.bowelcanceruk.org.uk/about-bowel-cancer/diagnosis/coping-with-diagnosis/.*

After my run, we tidy the house from top to bottom, and we're grateful to Emma's mum for assisting us with that. Today, our friends are visiting.

We trade family for friends, but we view them both as the same: our friends will spend the week with us, and we'll have some fun. I'll do my best to enjoy that fun while respecting my body and its needs.

Our friends arrive in the evening and, as we typically do, we meet at the pub. It's nice to go out for a drink, although I prefer not to have too many. They're also going through challenging times, and it's remarkable how simply having a conversation and sharing our feelings can be so helpful.

It's beneficial to talk, and as a man, I recognise the importance of doing it more – it's one of the purposes of these diaries.

Fellas, please talk.

31 December 2024

New Year's Eve. Honestly, I've never been a fan of New Year. It feels like forced fun. Instead of simply enjoying it, I feel pressured to follow the crowd and pretend to enjoy the day by dressing up, watching fireworks and singing a terrible song – goodness, I sound so miserable!

First, we go bowling with the crew. Our friends Michelle and Wayne and their children, Kelsie and Lucas, are staying with us. When I say children, I mean they're 21 and 17, respectively. Kelsie has brought her boyfriend, Owen, who joined us last year. We're amazed that he wants to join us again this year ☺ .

We're also joined by the lovely Issy and Frank, who have come to visit.

We go bowling and then curling. It's a lot of fun. I get two strikes in a row for the first time – maybe the tumour adds balance?

On our way home, we stop for a pint, then for another; after a few more drinks, we head home. We cook delicious food, chat, play games, and at ten past midnight, I go to bed. Everything is wrapped up as far as I'm concerned.

It's not going to be a happy New Year for me. It'll be a New Year where I focus on getting this thing out of me and then recovering. I hope my New Year begins on 1 February because that's when I expect to have recovered enough from the operation to function relatively normally. I also hope to have a plan moving forward from this date.

1 January 2025

I like to go out for a drink on New Year's Day, and today will be no different.

Knowing everyone is at home making resolutions and claiming they'll be healthy makes me want to do the opposite. I'm a quiet rebel, one of those people who actively avoids a box set or film if it's recommended to me. Sorry, everyone!

After a nice slow start to the day with a good breakfast prepared on my outdoor stove, we all go to our local pub. We planned to enjoy a long walk and drinks afterwards, but the weather is terrible.

Our local pub has a band playing. They're quite good, and we have such a lovely day. We all just sit chatting, discussing the year ahead, planning for our friend's wedding next year in Thailand – the things that help take your mind off what's happening in life. It's a good day, and I think it's one of the few days when I haven't thought about this treatment.

New Year – same me, no tumour.

2 January 2025

It's a lovely, bright winter day, a bit frosty and chilly, so we're taking the walk we missed yesterday.

Emma, our friends Wayne and Michelle, our two dogs, Norris and Frank, and I go for a lovely long walk through Reigate, Surrey.

We walk through farmers' fields and mud, enjoying it. It's something we all need. Today marks the first day of this festive period, and I feel somewhat off physically. My insides ache. While I'm not feeling great physically, I at least feel good mentally. It's lovely to be outside and breathe in the fresh air.

After our long walk, we meet Michelle and Wayne's kids, Kelsie, Lucas and Kelsie's boyfriend, Owen. We once again go to our local pub, share a couple of drinks, and have a good laugh. It's nice to engage in these activities and not think about what's ahead. This will be our last day with Michelle, Wayne and the kids, and tomorrow, reality begins to set in again.

3 January 2025

Once everyone leaves, this is the first day in a couple of weeks that no one else has been in the house. We wake up at around half past seven, meaning we've had over eight hours of sleep for the first time in a long while. The dogs are also sleeping. The house is quiet, and it feels good.

Today, we tackle the square root of nothing: we sort the laundry, and that's all we accomplish that feels productive. We check the cupboards to see how much Christmas food is still available and tidy up our stockings from the holiday. It's a lovely day as I catch up on some reading and continue writing these diary entries.

Physically, I feel pretty good today; each day seems different. I've still got pain in my side, but I think that's just my brain telling me it's there because I know the cancer is present. Mentally, I'm managing fairly well; I feel OK. I'm reading about positive thinking and simply trying to handle this situation properly.

I frequently reflect on my thoughts.

"This time in two weeks…"

"This time in two weeks…" and I can place myself in a better mental place by doing so.

4 January 2025

Today marks an exciting day for me as I'm off to enjoy watching Dorking Wanderers play.

I'm fortunate to have the opportunity to be a small shareholder in this wonderful club and also to serve as a sponsor. It's always a pleasant experience to go out and engage in something that feels normal and enjoyable, especially in today's world.

After making plans, we decide to meet up with my good friend Roger and his wonderful two children, Henry and Sam, who always bring joy to these outings.

Roger is familiar with facing difficult times in life. A couple of years ago, he encountered significant challenges that tested his strength. During our conversation, we reflect on those past difficulties and recall how life can unexpectedly throw obstacles in our way. Our main focus that day is to soak in the moment and enjoy the football match, hoping to escape the world's harsh realities temporarily. We settle in at the stadium, excited to cheer for Dorking Wanderers. The game ends with Dorking winning 1-0, which makes our day together even more special.

When the game finishes, we go back to Roger's to have dinner with him and his wife, Helen – my wife Emma's oldest friend. It's a lovely dinner.

We talk about what's coming, how we can support one another, and ultimately, how we hope that 2025 will turn out to be a good year, with my cancer and recovery being just a blip in the landscape.

5 January 2025

A quiet day begins with a run and ends with Liverpool drawing 2-2 with Manchester United.

I go for another run where I spend its entirety telling the cancer to go and fuck itself – sorry for the swearing; I write these diary entries in the moment and swearing sums up my mood today.

Reality is beginning to dawn. My mind keeps wandering, thinking about 'this time in a week', and I attempt to reprogramme it to 'this time in two weeks' when I'll better understand my progress and, hopefully, be back home.

6 January 2025

My first day back at work after Christmas and the day of my pre-operation assessment.

The pre-op was intense, filled with so much information and little brainpower to grasp what was happening. I can usually process a lot of information quickly, but today, I felt like I was in an alternate world where every word was a water-filled marigold slapping me across the face.

Appointment one was a health check in which they:

- Took my blood pressure
- Measured my height – I'm not 6 feet but they say I am
- Weighed me – I'll take 13 stone. Take that, BMI score!!
- Gave me an ECG
- Took 4 bottles of blood

I was also given:

- Antibiotics
- Bowel prep (laxatives) – joy
- Carb-loading drinks

Additionally, I received so much information about the operation and when and where I need to be. The nurse was so lovely and made a difficult situation much better!

Appointment two was with the Enhanced Recovery Nurse, who informed me about the operation. I'm having left-sided bowel surgery. We hope it'll be a keyhole procedure; however, it could require a full incision if they can't access my tumour. Oddly, she mentioned that my scars would be on the right side, and I had thought I'd be fine since I usually sleep on my right side.

Now, I'll have to sleep on my back; THAT'S A MAJOR SNORING POSITION.

Appointment three was with the Macmillan nurse, who will support me moving forward. We also discussed the possibility of having a stoma. I don't want a stoma, and they don't want to give me one, but I need to prepare for the possibility of having one – deep joy.

The whole afternoon was quite overwhelming. I left with so much printed information that it filled an entire tote bag. Furthermore, it knocked me for six; it made me realise this was real.

Until now, it felt like this was all happening to someone else; however, that no longer feels true.

It's happening to me, and I'm petrified.

7 January 2025

Today, I experienced a real wobble.

I was concerned about yesterday's visit to the hospital, talking to the nurses, wearing a mask, and doing all of this during a flu outbreak. Until now, it had almost felt like this was happening to someone else, but now it's happening to me.

In one week, I'll undergo surgery to have my bowel opened, repaired, or possibly removed, and I may awake with a stoma bag. All I can think about is how painful, annoying and scary this is.

All that said, I also have to realise that this time next week, my cancer will have been removed from me. I'll still need tests, and they'll still need to grade the tumour. But in essence, this lump in my bowel that has been giving me some grief will be gone, and I'll have a new challenge to recover, rest, recuperate and do what the doctors tell me, which won't be easy for me.

I'm also concerned about what will happen if I catch a cold or the flu. Being in that hospital yesterday and witnessing all those sick people wearing masks unsettled me. Thankfully, the nurses informed me that once the surgery is over, the ward I'll be in is separate from the main hospital and the corridors, making it significantly less likely for anyone with an illness to enter. Now, I've had to inform those planning to visit me that only one person can come at a time, and they need to wear a mask.

Understandably, they're now thinking, cripes, do I even want to go see him?

I went to bed feeling wobbly and consumed by worry; my mind felt heavy with concern. Although my sleep was less than restful, I drifted off for a while. Usually, I wake up at 5 am, but on this particular night, I stirred at 3:30 am and couldn't shake the feeling of unease; I recorded this diary entry at 4 am as I reflected on a night of broken dreams that haunted me.

These dreams were filled with vivid images of my tumour – the fear of pain gripping my thoughts like a vice. Each time I tried to return to sleep, I'd start worrying again; my dreams felt more like unsettling visions that left me feeling more anxious. In those dreams, I grappled with pain, my mind racing with questions about my health and what the future might hold. It was a restless night, with my body physically present in bed, yet my mind racing through a fog of dread and concern for what lay ahead.

This morning at around 7am, as I went to walk the dogs, I felt like I was about to burst into tears. However, during that walk, I told myself that no amount of negativity would help; I needed to be positive.

It feels so hard to be positive, but I have a word with myself.

I need to manifest positivity and abundant thinking.

As a side note, I want to thank Emma, Lucy, Suzy and Tara Swart for this. They're four amazing women who give me the strength to think clearly.

I need to realise that this cancer inside me is about to be removed. I need to realise that in a week, I'll be much more in control of my recovery than I have been at any point so far.

And during that week, all I have to do is follow the breathing exercises they taught me, attempt to get out of bed when it hurts, walk 60 metres four times a day, and, amusingly enough, fart.

That's right. F-A-R-T. I hope the word catches your attention.

Yes, if I fart, they'll let me leave the hospital as long as all my other 'vital' signs are fine. Luckily for me, farting ranks quite high on my top ten list of 'skills', and when I leave the hospital, I won't have to blame the dogs any more.

I resolve to practise farting over the next few days, as well as practising breathing and getting myself in the right mindset to tackle this and beat it.

Farts away. And oh yeah, fuck you, cancer!

A BOOK IS BORN. MY DECISION TO TELL THE WORLD.

8 January 2025

Today was a rather strange day. You see, unexpected things occurred that I had no idea were going to happen, and they were unrelated – yet at the same time, connected to the cancer.

I'm paranoid about getting a cold and anxious I'll fall ill before the operation, and it wasn't helped by the fact that I decided to call the nurses and ask if I could continue taking vitamins, and they told me no.

No to vitamins! I immediately feel like I'm on the back foot and out of control regarding my health.

My diet is low fibre, so I'm consuming very few fruits and vegetables. I'm eating very little of anything, which benefits me; it feels strange. I enjoy vegetables and like fruit occasionally. I don't want to continue eating beige food because I believe it might make me unwell, and now I'm concerned it could affect me before the operation, which is putting me in a heightened state of paranoia.

Eating low fibre isn't all bad, and it's necessary for my current health situation; if you're facing a similar predicament, you may find this information to be useful:

- *https://www.bowelcanceruk.org.uk/about-bowel-cancer/our-publications/eating-well/.*

A book is born. My decision to tell the world.

You can also find some incredible information on this page:

- *https://www.bowelcanceruk.org.uk/about-bowel-cancer/living-with-and-beyond-bowel-cancer/.*

I'm uncertain about what to do. I'm staying home, avoiding crowds, and only going out to walk the dogs, which is a pleasant distraction. Still, it's just that; in the back of my mind, the operation weighs heavily on me.

Will I be well? Will I be unwell?

Still, I remind myself that I need to think further ahead. Today, I can say that the operation should be finished by this time next week, and I anticipate that I'll be in charge of my recovery by this time next week.

Unfortunately, for me and Liverpool fans, Liverpool lost 0-1 this evening to Tottenham. But don't worry, we'll see you back at Anfield for the second leg in four weeks, and I hope to be fully recovered by then. My fingers are crossed.

I picture myself back home from hospital, watching the match, recovering and free of any cancerous tumour. I hope it turns out that way, along with a Liverpool win in the tie's second leg.

9 January 2025

Today is my last day with my client. I don't know when or even if I'll return.

Oddly, I'm still not worried about financial concerns. I must focus on surgery and recovery before I can think about that. My mind drifts to holidays; perhaps I'll have a six-pack for the beach…or a stoma. The stoma seems more likely.

A book is born. My decision to tell the world.

Packing up my desk and preparing my out-of-office still carries that 'holiday' vibe. Not that this is going to be a holiday at all.

10 January 2025

My worries about catching a cold persist. Last night, I went to bed early and rested for more than nine hours.

It's winter, and with temperatures at -2°C, hospitals across the nation are on high alert. The relentless cycle of doom and gloom in the news doesn't help, so finding sleep helps calm my mind.

Today, I choose to ignore the news and run a steady 25 minutes at 5 km, followed by an extra kilometre. This will be my last run before the operation and likely for quite some time. While at the gym, I once again see Wendy. Wendy is the lady who scheduled my colonoscopy. She's lovely and wishes me luck for Monday.

I have a thought as I run: writing these diary entries daily has proved to be cathartic. When I return home, I read them back and find it interesting that the feelings I've experienced have been so mixed. I also wonder whether they could help others.

I've written two books and co-authored another in my professional life. If you've read one of my books and this diary, you'll see how hard my copy editors work!

In the case of two of my books, my writing is less from the heart and more based on my working life, but it's when thinking about this that I realise these experiences could be worth sharing.

A book is born. My decision to tell the world.

After chatting with Emma, I create a Substack and compile my diary entries into it. That afternoon flies by, and it's where this book is born. What began as a Substack should now be a book in your hands. I write these words today, hoping to manifest a book and an audiobook.

As I embark on this journey, I envision a publisher recognising the potential of my work. I hope they'll perceive the passion and sincerity within the pages, motivating them to pick it up and help share it with a broader audience. The idea of a traditional publisher supporting this project thrills me, as it would validate my efforts and allow my stories to connect with even more readers.

I'm determined to give back. I plan to donate some of the profits to charity because my work should help others. It's essential to me that this book not only fulfils my creative ambitions but also contributes positively to the world.

By supporting a charity that aligns with the themes of my writing, I hope to make a meaningful impact. Every turned page could make a difference to another person, and that's a hopeful vision I hold for this endeavour.

If you're reading this, then I will have been proved correct.

As I sit here preparing to hit 'publish' this afternoon, I can't help but feel a wave of anxiety wash over me. Announcing this on LinkedIn isn't just a casual update; it's an unsettling experience filled with uncertainty and self-reflection.

I find myself struggling with a series of questions:

Am I attracting unnecessary attention?

Am I sharing this with genuine intent?

A book is born. My decision to tell the world.

Or am I driven by something less admirable?

The fear of judgement looms large in my mind, particularly concerning how potential clients will perceive my words.

What if they see my post and think less of me? What if they draw incorrect conclusions about my expertise or character based on a few lines of text? It's nerve-wracking because our professional identities are often tied to how we present ourselves publicly. I start to rationalise my feelings, trying to mitigate the fear with logical reassurance. I remind myself, "If a prospective client doesn't appreciate what I have to say, then that's really their problem, not mine." Yet, deep down, I know that sharing this is a leap of faith that could either foster connections or provoke criticisms that I'm not sure I'm ready to face.

In these moments of self-doubt, I reflect on the balance between vulnerability and strength. I question my professionalism, wondering whether my desire to communicate is worth the risks it entails. Putting myself out there is inherently unsettling; however, it's a necessary step in building an authentic presence and reaching those who might genuinely resonate with my thoughts and insights.

However, I'm often confident, and while sitting here thinking about publishing my writing, I find that I'm not focused on cancer. This writing and sharing my story gives me a sense of purpose, so I decide to go for it and publish this diary for the 'world' to see.

I truly hope someone reads this diary and finds help in it. We men don't talk enough, and I'm hopeful that my writing will assist others while also helping me.

Within 24 hours, my LinkedIn post gets 15,000 views, 70 comments and over 130 reactions. My Substack has more than 300 reads and 36 new subscribers. Wow!

Numbers do not drive me, but I hope these numbers justify my decision.

Thank you to everyone.

11 January 2025

I woke up today after not getting the best night's sleep. I tend to wake up during the night for about five minutes. During those five minutes, I try to forget what's coming, and when I can't ignore it, I remind myself to be grateful for my surgery; in only a few days, this cancer inside me will be removed. After that, it's up to me to focus on my physical health and recovery, as well as continue working on my mental health, which is something this diary helps with.

My day begins with a shower using a flannel and some shower gel provided by the hospital. It's a clear liquid that I must spread all over myself; it's somewhat smelly and stings my eyes; it appears that my world of pain has started two days early.

Emma and I are having a really quiet day; my paranoia about catching a cold persists, although it doesn't stop us from taking the dogs out for a walk in -6°C. The dogs love it, and as we walk around on this sunny winter's day, I think to myself how fortunate I am to have a roof over my head, a bed to sleep in, an incredible wife, two wonderful dogs,, who give me 35 to 40 minutes of joy as we stroll through these snowy fields.

And so, we hunker down for the day as Liverpool plays in the FA Cup against Accrington Stanley ("WHO ARE THEY? EXACTLY," IYKYK). Liverpool wins 4-0, and Accrington don't disgrace themselves. I'm very happy with that result.

This is also when I'm eating more beige food, so I settle down for a veggie sausage sandwich, an egg custard tart and some leftover pizza from last night. However, I have to remove the onions, peppers and mushrooms – essentially all the vegetables. If I haven't mentioned this before, it's crazy that I'm on the least healthy diet I've ever had right before major surgery.

We watch a Netflix series called *La Palma*. It's intriguing. It depicts how a tsunami that could devastate the Americas and the Canary Islands might occur if La Palma were to plunge into the sea.

I've discovered a new comedy on Disney+ that I highly recommend. It's called *Dave*. Although I dislike being called Dave, I enjoy this comedy because the word makes me laugh.

We go to bed, and I hear Emma's phone rumbling throughout the night, but I know it's nothing urgent. I'm part of a WhatsApp group with Emma and our friends from my hometown of Congleton, and I know they're in their kitchens having a boogie, chatting about music and discussing plans. It's quite reassuring to listen to it buzz, buzz, buzz until about two in the morning. It's nice to know that others are having a good time.

One thing I've tried to maintain is a feeling that just because I'm in a shit situation, I shouldn't let envy or jealousy overtake me. Life goes on, and I truly hope that it goes on faultlessly and with love and laughter for everyone else. We'll be back there on WhatsApp and out with friends, reflecting on this moment and thinking about a bright future.

12 January 2025

Before I write today's diary entry, what I have to do today is listed below. All to prep for surgery.

- 08:00 Take antibiotics/shower and wash my hair in the rancid liquid
- 12:00 More antibiotics
- 14:00 First MoviPrep (laxative) bowel treatment
- 16:00 Hospital-provided carb drink
- 17:00 More antibiotics
- 18:00 Second MoviPrep bowel treatment
- 20:00 Second hospital-provided carb drink
- And if it's helpful today, I eat:
  - 09:00 Toast, butter and shredless marmalade (white bread)
  - 13:00 A sandwich on white bread, a custard tart
  - 17:30 Chicken and rice, literally just chicken and white rice

We take the boys for another lovely morning walk. I won't do this for six weeks, so I savour every moment.

I download some shows to my iPad, an offline version of this diary, along with a lot of music. Since I love listening to music, I get my favourite artists, DJs and stations through Mixcloud and create a Spotify playlist.

I pack underwear, T-shirts, toiletries, my first pair of pyjamas and my first dressing gown; I've never had PJs or a dressing gown before – is that too much info?

Finally, we settle down and watch *The Great Pottery Throw Down* while I take calls from friends and family wishing me well and drink my final carb drink. We then go to bed at 9:45 pm and set an alarm for 5:25 am.

Next stop: Surgery

EMMA'S BIRTHDAY AND THE SURGERY

13 January 2025

Today is Emma's birthday, and it's surgery day.

I wake at 3:51 am. My Oura Ring tells me I slept 5 hours and 33 minutes. I'm happy with that; my Oura Ring also indicates that it took me 15 minutes to fall asleep. Bonus.

It's Emma's birthday, and I'm determined she will enjoy some of today. After I showered with the antiseptic wash and prepared my final carb drink, we lay in bed and opened Emma's presents from me. In truth, they're tokens, and we plan to celebrate her birthday when this is all done.

One item is broken, which is frustratingly typical. Em says she doesn't want to worry about her birthday, but I find it deeply unfair that today has to be about me and not her.

I'll make up for it.

We leave home at 6:35 and check in for pre-surgery admissions at 7 am. Over the next few hours, I meet with the surgeons and the anaesthetist and have my blood drawn before sitting in a very uncomfortable chair from which I write this entry.

I also have the stoma stickers applied as a precaution.

I joke with the surgeon that all my wife wants for her birthday is a cancer-free husband, one with as much bowel as possible and no stoma – mainly so she doesn't have to hear me moan about it. He laughs and promises to do his very best; I trust him.

At around 11:30 am, I'm called to follow a lady up to the top floor, where I change into a gown and sit/lie in a sterile room for an hour. I'm nervous but not panicking, which surprises me; I keep thinking, "You've come this far."

While there, I overhear a heartbreaking moment: a lady is there due to an emergency; she's had a miscarriage and needs surgery. I hear her and her partner sobbing, and I lie there feeling so sorry for them. I'm having something removed that I never wanted; they have an entirely more heartbreaking and soul-destroying predicament to deal with.

I hope you both feel better now and plan for a brighter future.

Next, I'm collected and wheeled into a sterile room that feels cold and unwelcoming. The bright lights overhead cast a harsh glare, intensifying my anxiety as I see the anaesthetists moving around, preparing for the operation. I notice the large screens in the operating theatre and immediately get a flashback to seeing my tumour during the colonoscopy. I know that my insides will be displayed on those screens in just a few minutes.

I feel a knot tightening in my stomach as I try to focus on their calm demeanour, telling myself they do this daily. Like it or not, I've come this far, and there's no going back. I wonder if the tightening is my tumour, sensing its time is almost up!

They begin preparing me for the operation, starting with an injection in my back. Despite my racing heart, I engage in small talk, sharing stories about my tattoos – a feeble attempt to distract myself from the overwhelming situation. I know this is intended to ease my nerves, but inside, I grapple with a chaotic mix of fear and acceptance, struggling to find solace as I surrender to their expertise and the reality of what's about to happen.

Then, I'm instructed to arch my back; this is where my 'real' anaesthetic is directed. I can't lie – it hurts a little, but it's not too bad. (It's bloody excruciating.)

I'm then laid on my back, asked how I feel, and have machines attached to me. Next, I'm instructed to inhale gas and count to ten.

1-2-3 lights out.

13 January 2025 – Emma's Birthday and the surgery

I can't remember the operation. This is the only time I've had to 'write' in my diary the day after the events. Truthfully, this entry was spoken into my phone, and it took me some time to tidy it up. My voice slurred, and my thought process was interrupted by morphine.

I come to, I think, five hours later in recovery, and I have a wonderful nurse. My first action is to reach to my left side; however, I can't feel anything.

I literally can't feel anything. I'm numb.

"You don't have a stoma," says the nurse.

Thank FUCK, I say to myself.

I also ask if Emma can see me tonight. The answer is no, but she knows I've undergone the surgery and come out the other side.

Happy Birthday, babe.

The nurse is lovely, and by the end of our chat over the next hour, I've convinced her to sign up for my Substack. She's teaching someone, and I appreciate watching a skilled teacher who offers empathy, experience and a constructive critique. She's a good teacher; I tell her this when her student leaves her.

I'm taken to the ward, and that night feels somewhat hazy.

What I do know is that I'm managing to fart, which, for me, is fantastic since I know it's something I have to do before I leave the hospital; that's one thing to check off.

And when I say fart, I mean Faaaaaaaarrrrrrrrrttttttt – riproaring, earth-shuddering farts. I even catch the nurse laughing.

The night is a blend of beeping machines, morphine available via a button, and getting acclimatised to the environment.

At midnight, I begin to vomit, as I fully expected I would. I don't recover from the anaesthetic very well, and even though they're giving me drugs to help, I can't help but projectile vomit without knowing how to contact the nurse. I think it's a mixture of the drugs and not being told where the button is. So, I grab one of the 'pee hats' and throw up in that – so dignified. Now I'm farting and throwing up at the same time; oddly, I chuckle to myself. I think it's the morphine.

I really enjoy the morphine; I've used it 67 times, primarily to help me sleep, but also because I'm listening to some rave music that fits my mood.

I'm lying there watching the walls dance to my music and loving it.

14 January 2024 – The recovery begins

I wake up while having my blood taken at 5 am and having my catheter removed; oh, that was a pain. It's a real shooting pain; I invite you to try it one day.

At 7 am, as the shift changes, the strangest thing happens. I recognise the 'day' nurse. It's Julie, a lady I often drink with at my local pub. Immediately, I worry about this situation. What if Julie sees my bits and bobs? What if I'm sick? What will Julie think of me?

I decide there's only one way to handle this. "Alright, Julie," I croak from my bed. At first, she doesn't recognise me, but then, upon realisation, Julie comes in and says, "Hi," and asks me how I am. Julie returns to her rounds, but not before I ask her if they serve Guinness on the ward.

The Enhanced Recovery team visit me at my bedside after breakfast. I devour breakfast – it's just yoghurt, but I always say it's the most important meal. I'm unsure if I should even feel hungry, but I do, and it makes me happy.

The Enhanced Recovery team attempts to get me out of bed, and I feel extremely dizzy. It's to be expected, though they don't make a big issue of it, and I get back into bed. It's here that I realise I have a very numb left leg – so numb that I can't feel my knee or the surrounding area.

I meet with the surgeon, who tells me that he removed a tumour the size of a half-fist, but he also mentions that it hadn't perforated the bowel, although he did notice a couple of enlarged lymph nodes nearby. That's all I need to know from there.

At 11 am, Emma comes to visit me. I believe she feels relieved to see me. She hasn't seen me since she left me in preparation for the operation yesterday, on her birthday. I tell her that I'm feeling fine, but I think I'm a bit loopy from the morphine, though not nearly as bad as I was last night.

Evidence provided below. PS Fox's Glacier Mints are my go-to when hungover, and a top tip (from me) after bowel resection.

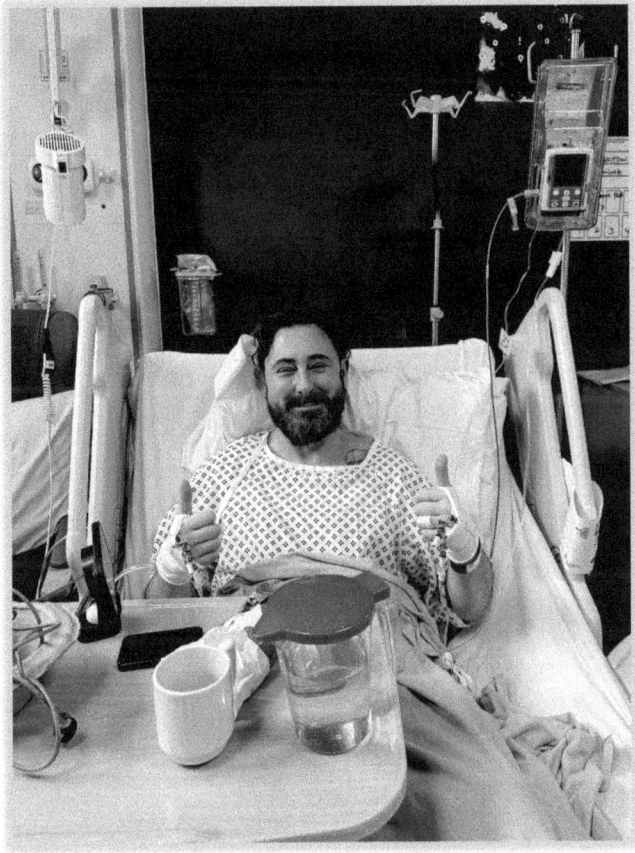

Post-Op Morphine Smiles

Emma fills me in on how her birthday was. It sounds like the worst birthday she could have had – just people asking about me and waiting for me to come out of the theatre, only to be told it was too late to visit. We'll make up for it one day.

By midday, I start to feel stronger as the anti-sickness drugs take effect. I begin to eat, and as I eat, I feel energy returning to me – my father comes to visit, which is lovely considering he's travelled so far. He's driven 240 miles to spend time with me; I'm not sure I make any sense as we chat.

I also spend that time drinking jug after jug of water in an attempt to 'naturally' go for a pee. After a few failed attempts, it finally comes, and it's a huge relief because I know this is another box ticked in my recovery. I feel awful as I ask poor Julie to take away my pee to be sampled. I'm embarrassed and ashamed, but Julie reassures me it's fine and smiles as I suggest I will get her a different kind of drink the next time I see her.

I also take this time to get out of bed because I can't pee while lying down; once again, I notice that my knee is completely numb.

After a few hours, Dad and Emma let me rest.

I choose not to rest; I want to rise. I take it upon myself to start my recovery. I get out of bed and head towards Julie. "Can I go for a walk?" Julie says yes, and we joke that I might not make it as far as the pub while Julie shows me how to push my IV down the ward.

I take a few laps around the ward with my morphine, which, incidentally, I haven't touched in quite a while. Getting up and moving is beneficial, and I can move my legs, although the left one remains numb.

The doctors are concerned that some anaesthetic might be trapped in my left knee. I'm not certain, but I can feel the stomach pain returning. I request to have my surgical stockings removed from the affected leg, and it provides some relief.

That night, I'm back in bed watching Liverpool draw 1-1 with Nottingham Forest. I'm exhausted but still can't sleep. It's bright, it isn't quiet, and I really don't know how I'm going to drift off. Suddenly, I wake up at 2 am, get up, go to the loo, and wake up again at 5:15 am for a blood test – job done.

Recovery Day 1 boxed off.

For those wondering about the pain, it's not great, but I think I can manage with paracetamol and ibuprofen by the evening. As a result, we remove the morphine line – goodbye my friend.

15 January 2025

A day filled with surprises.

Surprise one: I amaze the nurses and doctors by completing 1,000 steps by 9 am. I'm not doing this to appear impressive or brave, nor to present myself as something I'm not. I'm doing it because I understand how important it is to keep moving after surgery.

I still can't feel my left knee. We're not sure whether it's anaesthesia or possibly the bed that's preventing me from feeling it. Still, I know that by moving around and making my leg work by rotating my hip, I can feel my knee again, and I can feel it improving already, which is great.

Surprise two: These walks take me past the reception desk, where the nurses, doctors, cleaner, tea lady work. I chat with them as I pass by, discussing various topics while I wander. I also converse with the ward sister, who is a poet and songwriter.

We discuss her exceptional talent and passion; she's amazing. Originally from Grenada, she has written songs and poems about her homeland, as well as about her experiences as a nurse, which she shares with me. They're wonderful. She works in the medical profession, while I work in IT. I've published three books, but she is a far better writer than I am. She shows me her songs and poetry. Later, I gave her a copy of my recently co-authored book with Lucy, which I brought to read. You may wonder why; well, writing a book is peculiar in that when you write it, you read it in segments, and I think I'd like to read it as a whole.

The book is called *Allyship Actually*. I write, "TO PATRICIA, FOLLOW YOUR DREAMS." I think I see a tear as she looks through the book.

Surprise three: I have amazed the specialists with my recovery. I may be able to go home tomorrow, Thursday. The specialist and I discuss my mental outlook when she notices I've been reading *The Source*. She mentions that if all patients adopted my mindset, more people would recover and recuperate quickly.

First and foremost, there are certain conditions for my leaving tomorrow. I must continue taking blood tests, including measuring my blood pressure and temperature, because there are aspects that no patient can deceive about, but so far, I'm doing really, really well.

I also need to keep moving around to get my knee functioning properly. It's a mixture of a dead leg and pins and needles. It feels strange as I move about, but I'm sure it's due to the bed. When I massage the lower left-hand side of my back, I notice a bit of swelling. It's sore. I think I've trapped a nerve, and it seems to be transmitting pain into my leg. I explain this to the specialist, and she says I'm probably onto something, but they'll send the anaesthetist up later.

When the anaesthetist arrives, she tells me they think the anaesthetic injected into my spine may be the cause. She apologises, but when I mention the bed, she says we shouldn't blame the beds. However, she acknowledges I might have a point, so if you ever go into the hospital for surgery, I must tell you the beds aren't comfortable.

They have many adjustable settings, but not one hits the word 'comfortable'. They're just varying degrees of discomfort. I'm sure they've got good medical uses, but believe me, they're not suitable for sleeping on.

Surprise four: Kipster. My father visits me in the morning.

We have a small problem.

We discovered just yesterday that each patient is allowed one visitor per day. The hospital is concerned about norovirus and the seasonal flu, which is exactly what I was so anxious about last week.

I've managed to secure a visit for my dad, who is coming from Manchester. They understand that my wife wants to see me, so in my brief conversations with the front desk, I've arranged for both visits under strict orders that they wear masks and keep their stay brief. After Dad leaves, as far as I'm concerned, Emma is coming to see me.

Then, arriving in the doorway and screaming **"SURPRISE!"** is Kipster, aka Kip, or sometimes known by his real name, Paul. He bursts into the room and once again exclaims, "SURPRISE!"

He flew from Spain this morning to see me and is flying back this afternoon. It's such a great tonic to see him. Even though I'm scared they're going to kick him out, he stays. Fortunately, none of the nurses bother us, even when Kip steps out and asks them where the nearest vending machine is. Never change, mate.

We chat. He makes me laugh, and I realise that laughing hurts. It's so kind of him to come and so nice to see him, even though I'm sitting in a gown feeling as rough as badgers the whole time he's there.

Thanks, Kipster.

PS I gave the chocolates to the nurses, as they told me I couldn't eat them – it's the thought that counts.

I also realise that engaging with people and being present can be quite challenging. I'm exhausted, possibly more tired than I've ever been. I feel lethargic yet also filled with joy that my friend has travelled such a distance to see me. All I want to do is sleep tonight and recover from this operation.

And then, thanks to my speedy recovery, they move me from a room to a ward.

Eeesh.

This evening's plans to fall asleep are slowly falling apart because I've made such a good recovery. The nurses would like to take my room and offer it to someone else who needs it.

I have no problems with that, and I readily agree to move into the ward opposite. When I toddle over, I find a poor man in the middle of the ward, not even in his own bay, as all the other bays are full.

Each of us has undergone some form of surgery in the last few days. None of us is worse off than the others, nor does any of us deserve any better treatment. But believe me, watching people attempt to urinate in paper bottles with their bare bottoms exposed, and in some cases, their penises on display while sharing a toilet with a bunch of strangers, makes me long for that room back.

Additionally, the ward smells terrible. Just what you'd expect from a ward filled with men dealing with post-operative bowel and bladder issues, and the sounds – oh, the sounds – are something else entirely; it's as if a whoopee cushion contest has erupted.

Tonight, I settle into my uncomfortable bed and try to get some sleep. I listen to audiobooks and music while wearing a blindfold. I do everything I can to sleep but can't manage it. It's how I find myself adding to today's diary during the evening.

My neighbour is snoring the place down. Directly opposite me I can only see the private parts of a very confused man and next to him is a gentleman who I later learn has unfortunately strained too hard and pushed outside what should be inside, and every time he bends over to tuck it up,

I get a full view as it catches the lights on the ward. My heart goes out to him.

To avoid these noises and views, I spend the night walking up and down the ward, going back to bed, going to the loo, and doing my best to maintain a positive mindset. This amounts to over 5,000 steps.

16 January 2025

Last night was the hardest I've had in a while; it's the reality of hospital life. It has made it difficult for me to maintain my positive attitude, but all I can think about is the potential to leave the hospital today. It's this that motivates me to keep going.

Typically, I finally fell asleep at around 4 am, only to be awakened at 5:15 am by the nurse taking my blood pressure and temperature. However, a part of me felt quite happy as I checked my pulse rate, which was 62.

This indicates that I'm relaxed, which should hopefully aid me in my quest to exit the building. All I need to worry about now is my blood tests. So far, they've all been good, and I hope they continue to be. Fingers crossed!

I experience some pain when I go to the loo from where my catheter was placed. A catheter is a thin, flexible tube inserted into the body to drain fluids or deliver medication. In a post-operative context, catheters are often used to help patients manage urinary function after surgery, especially if they're unable to urinate independently.

Proper catheter placement and care are essential to prevent complications like infections or blockages. Although mine was removed a day or two ago, I want to ensure it hasn't caused any issues. I'm doing my best to take control of the situation. I ask the nurse if she can test my urine, and she agrees. I want to make sure I've covered all bases before the surgeon and specialist see me later today, except for sleep. I spend the next 45 minutes drinking water before giving my sample to the nurse.

Thankfully (meant in the nicest possible way), it's not Julie overnight.

By 6 am, I'm back in the chair next to my bed, trying to fall asleep while watching YouTube and reading.

There's one thing that could keep me in the hospital – my bile bag. It's attached to my stomach where my main puncture site is, and it's collecting my blood; I'm told it's also gathering the serum they infused into my body during the operation. At some point, it's supposed to stop filling, but looking down, I see it hanging by my thigh, two-thirds full and showing no signs of stopping – what a pain, quite literally.

Even if I could, I'm not going to insist they remove it because it's doing some good. Indeed, when the specialist in the team of doctors comes around, they look at it and say they want me to stay in for another 24 hours. Please, no!

Now let me help you picture the scene.

I grimly smile as I tell the specialist, "I don't like you any more."

She laughs. She understands what I mean. I explain that last night, I got only one hour and 40 minutes of sleep, and I need to rest in order to recover from this operation. I'm doing everything else they're asking of me, including the blood tests and blood-pressure checks, not to mention my urine tests, the results of which I obviously can't fake, and they're telling the medical staff that I'm doing well.

With this, the Enhanced Recovery Nurse speaks up and says, "David is way ahead of schedule." The specialist then turns to me and says, "How far away do you live?"

I explain that it's barely five minutes in the car and plead with her that I'll return every day if necessary.

"BRILLIANT," she says. "Come back tomorrow, and we'll check that bag; hopefully, we can remove it then."

And so begins my escape. Firstly, I need to empty this bag and strap it to my leg instead of letting it hang off me; it's not nice.

Earlier today, I managed to have a really good wash and change into some fresh pyjamas, which feels nice, apart from the bag hanging from me. I also need to collect 26 injections that I'll have to self-administer.

I immediately ask the nurse why I need these, as no one had informed me about them before the operation, and I had been quite looking forward to some time without needles.

The nurse explains that post-operative blood thinners, also known as anticoagulants, play a crucial role in preventing blood clots in patients after surgery. These clots can lead to serious complications, such as deep vein thrombosis (DVT) or pulmonary embolism, which can be life-threatening. After surgery, mobility may be limited, increasing the likelihood of clot formation. Blood thinners reduce this risk by inhibiting blood from clotting, promoting better circulation and supporting overall heart health.

I think it's important to include this in the diary, as I hope it helps you or a friend understand how this works. It can significantly aid in recovery and reduce the risk of post-operative complications. That said, I remind the nurse that no one informed me of this, and I ask, "Can't I just take aspirin?"

She laughs it off, and while we chat, I devise a cunning plan and tell them that Emma will do it. So, when Emma comes in, she has to be shown how to do it. Emma, as is her way, doesn't flinch; she takes everything in her stride and is as amazing as ever – my rock!

I'm covered in tattoos, but I'm scared of needles. Even after going through all the injections, blood tests and everything else they've done to me, I can't think of anything worse than injecting myself. So, I trust Emma to do it.

And with that, I'm out of the hospital at half past one in the afternoon. It's been barely 72 hours since my operation, and it feels so good to get that fresh air. I waddle to the car, climbing in and placing the pillow that Emma brought over my stomach, and we drive home.

Every bump in the road hurts. Every bump in the road reminds me that only 72 hours ago, I had part of my bowel removed to eliminate a tumour, and each reminder makes me smile. I won't say I'm cancer-free, but I'm one step closer to being cancer-free and also closer to recovery.

When we get home, our window cleaner is outside. I also know him quite well. He drinks at my local pub and shouts over, "What's going on with you?" Rather than lie, I explain that I've just had a bowel operation for cancer.

He asks me when it was, and when I say Monday, he responds, "Fuck me, you look incredible for someone who had a bowel operation three days ago."

I laugh (it hurts), thank him, and tell him I'll see him in a couple of weeks, hopefully at the pub. Our window cleaner is named Luis. He's a lovely, cheerful man, and before I leave, he tells me, "If you need anything, you've got my number. Anything at all, I'll bring it over."

Luis's small gesture reminds me that I've been truly blessed during this treatment to have so many kind people around me, and it reassures me that we, as humans, are not as bad as the news and politicians would have us believe.

When I get home, the dogs go crazy. Poor Emma has to restrain them with their leads, but slowly, we let them sniff me until they eventually calm down. Being back with my boys is bliss.

I walk around the house deciding which bed I'll sleep in since I have to stay in a room without the dogs. After all, they enjoy jumping up on the bed. I choose our largest spare room and laugh as I struggle to get in and out of bed. After finally settling down, I try to relax for a few hours. By now, it's 4 pm, and at 7 pm, Emma will need to give her first injection into my leg – something neither of us is looking forward to.

After the injection, which goes well, I settle back into bed. I'm so tired that I worry I won't sleep, so I play relaxing music, take paracetamol and a sleeping tablet, and drift off.

17 January 2025

Last night, I slept for almost ten hours – the best sleep I've had since December.

I had some good sleep before the operation, but it wasn't restful. This sleep feels different. It feels like it's helping me recover and move forward. Finally, I feel like I'm on the road to recovery.

I wake up at 5 am – the good thing is that I always wake up at 5 am. I struggle to get myself comfy in bed, but I laugh as I do so. I look down and see that my bag is still full of juice. I say to myself, "I don't think this will be removed today," and I make peace with it.

Emma kindly prepares me a lovely peppermint tea, which I've been told is very beneficial for my digestive system. It seems to be effective. My bowels are perhaps 50% of what they used to be, but they're getting better.

While Emma walks the dogs, I get up and take the best wash possible. I've wanted to do this since Tuesday morning, and it feels wonderful. I eat a bagel with honey and enjoy a fresh coffee. Emma manages all this while dealing with two excited dogs before and after the walk.

Once I'm dressed, Emma heads to the gym, and I recline. I check all the messages that people have sent me.

Thank you. If you are reading this and have sent me a message, you brought me smiles throughout the treatment. You reassured me that people are good, and I'll thank you for that when I see you one day.

The great escape

Emma and I head to the hospital at 11 am to see my specialist, Sara, who allowed me to leave yesterday. Typically, she's busy, and it's 1:15 pm before she can get to us again. I'm not bothered. I might be sitting in a room with people sniffing and coughing, but I've got a mask on, and I'm just chilling.

When I see her, I watch her clock the bag. She says it's still filling up, so we can't take it out today. Sara shows me how to clean and empty it. I'll return on Tuesday to have it removed, when she's back at work, and hopefully, it'll have stopped filling up.

Yes, it's awkward, and I don't like having it on me. Yes, it makes sleeping difficult, but yes, I'm back home and ready to continue this recovery.

In the evening, Emma makes pasta that may seem simple, but it's the most substantial meal I've had since last Saturday. Earlier, Emma and I discussed how it seems I've lost weight in my face. I look gaunt, and my eyes appear unfamiliar. I haven't lost weight in my belly, as it's still swollen and bruised from the operation, but when I look into my eyes, I can sense that I have a long path to recovery ahead of me.

My energy levels aren't what they used to be, but that pasta is fantastic. For those of you reading this, it's that pasta that allowed me to write this just before going to sleep; it provided the energy boost I needed.

The only problem with eating pasta is that my stomach doesn't appreciate it as much as my mouth does. Part of this recovery involves relearning what I can and can't eat. Later on, I feel absolutely terrible, and my stomach hurts. I have pain rattling around my digestive system; I can feel it moving about. I can't get comfortable, which makes sleeping difficult. I suppose that's the issue with surgery: you need to relearn what you can and can't cope with physically, mentally, and internally.

All that said, it's nice to be home. It's nice to relax and get comfortable, and frankly, it's nice to fart without worrying that four other people in the room can hear you.

Here are my takeaways from the surgery

Number one: You don't need to pack a great deal. I packed three pairs of pants, three pairs of socks, three T-shirts, a tracksuit and one pair of pyjamas. I wore one pair of pyjamas, and that was on the last day.

I packed a wash bag full of items I didn't need. Everything I required was at the hospital, but I suggest you bring a wash bag – just in case.

Number two: Maintaining a positive mental attitude is the difference between leaving the hospital quickly and being stuck there. The nurses, doctors, oncologists and specialists could see that I was determined to manage my recovery, but I did so in a way that allowed me to smile with them, talk with them and listen to their advice. I honestly believe that if I hadn't approached it this way, I might still be in the hospital until Tuesday of the following week.

It also helps to live nearby.

Number three: Morphine is great, but they monitor how much you take. I quickly noticed that they checked the numbers every time they came to see me, so I asked them, "Do you know how much morphine I'm taking?"

The answer was yes, so I took the morphine when I needed it, but I didn't use it to help me sleep. If I wasn't in pain, I didn't take it. This means I stopped the morphine by Tuesday afternoon. I was also off the intravenous paracetamol by Wednesday morning, and now I'm just taking paracetamol and ibuprofen. Let's see how that goes.

Number four: Taking their advice and getting out of bed to move as soon as possible is beneficial. The first time I got out of bed, I felt lightheaded, sat down, and they put me back to bed. They were encouraging and told me I had done the right thing, but I felt disappointed.

Getting back out of bed when I could was the correct choice. Walking around was the right decision. It gets you moving and activates your muscles, and I can feel the difference after a few days. However, it didn't excuse me from the freaking blood-thinning injections.

Number five: Hospitals are not easy places to sleep. They always have to check on you, and as a result, they're constantly checking on everyone else, which means there's always someone walking around doing something while you're trying to sleep. My advice is to bring a sleep mask, a good book, and anything else that helps you rest because you'll need it.

Don't let that discourage you. They're taking care of you; they're measuring aspects you could never hope to assess on your own, and by doing so, they'll enhance your outcome.

Number six: Hospital food isn't great, but they're doing their best with limited resources, and I want to thank them for that. For now, these are my key takeaways from being in the hospital. Aside from being experts, they're well-studied and know what they're doing, so please trust them to handle it well.

And so, here I am on a Friday evening, writing this diary entry, reflecting on the past week. I had thought to myself that perhaps the worst would be over by next week, yet here we are, a week later.

Yes, I'm in pain. Yes, I have a bag hanging from me, but is it as bad as I thought it would be?

Honestly, I don't believe it is.

The pain is uncomfortable, and the bag is certainly painful, but I no longer have a tumour inside me, so I consider that a win.

This Friday evening, I watch TV, enjoy a few squares of Dairy Milk, sip an ice-cold Ribena, and have Emma inject blood thinners into my leg.

And I'm thankful for all of those things.

IN PAIN AND FEELING MARGINALISED

18 January 2025

It's arguably the most boring day ever. Today, I choose to follow the doctor's orders and rest as much as possible.

I lie in bed all day, only getting up occasionally to go to the loo, stretch my legs and wander around. I catch up with my dad and friends and have good conversations over FaceTime with those who want to know how I'm doing and about my recovery.

With nothing to do, I spend some time researching bile bags, specifically the one currently hanging from my stomach. I'm desperately trying to understand whether it's a good or a bad thing. In the end, after Doctor Google scares the life out of me, I decide it's not for me to understand; it's up to the doctors.

Today is Dorking Wanderers' 1000th game, and I'm unable to attend for obvious reasons, but I do get to watch the game online. I spend the afternoon with Dorking on one iPad and Liverpool v Brentford on the other screen. Sadly, Dorking loses, but Liverpool wins 2-0 with goals in the 91st and 93rd minutes, which makes my day.

I find that cheering really hurts! Go on, Darwin, lad!

Watching Arsenal surrender a two-goal lead against Aston Villa makes my day even better. I apologise for the constant football references if you're reading this and aren't into football. For me, having a distraction, being able to watch my team perform well, and enjoying around 90 minutes not thinking about cancer, the operation, the pain, or even the bag hanging from my stomach on my leg is truly wonderful.

I have soup for dinner this evening – not really what I'd prefer on a 'usual' Saturday, but it seems sensible. At least, I think so until I find myself rolling around in pain at about 10 pm, wondering what the hell is going on. The pain is excruciating.

I'm gradually learning to discern whether the pain is muscular or internal. This pain is internal, relating to my colon being resectioned. It doesn't concern me; I take ibuprofen and drift off to sleep.

19 January 2025

I wake up after six hours of sleep – not as much as I'd like, but good sleep, nonetheless. However, today is a day that begins with a surprise. Apologies if you're squeamish or if this is too much detail, but I wake up and have a massive solid number two.

You need to understand that when I was informed about the operation, I was told I might never regain my normal bowel movements. It could take weeks, months, years, or possibly longer to wake up, have a mint tea, and then think, maybe I should pop to the toilet. That was one of the most pleasant surprises of my experience.

What a way to start the Sabbath! After that, I have nothing to report – just recovery.

20 January 2025

It's another night of poor sleep. It seems that every time I go to bed, my stomach turns and flips, and I knot myself up in anxiety. I'm not sure what it is, but I ate six hours before bed today and felt no pain until I tried to sleep.

I had a sleepy hot chocolate before bed and wondered if that could be the cause.

Anyway, I fell asleep after taking some painkillers and managed to rest for five hours and 18 minutes. It wasn't the best night's sleep, but it was still much better than the one hour or so I got in the hospital last week.

Because I haven't slept much, I start the day in a more leisurely way than I should, sipping mint tea in bed while watching last night's TV. Yet, as I sit there, I feel frustrated.

I want to go for a run, and at that moment, when I see someone running past the house, I think my bag of blood and I are going to go out.

Incidentally, today marks the first day I've observed a decrease in blood, bile or whatever is in that bag. That's good news.

So, I put on my coat and trainers, neither of which is as easy as it once was, and I walk 0.6 km around the block. Getting the fresh air is lovely, but it's tough.

I laughed before the operation, thinking, how tough could it be? I routinely run 5 km or 10 km; I ran 50 km last year, yet 0.6 km feels almost as hard as my ultramarathon last year.

Today felt even more challenging. However, I believe this is the first step towards my next ultramarathon, and I've already got my eye on one.

Today marks one week post-op; the nightmare appears to be fading into the distance.

It also seems to be the case when people write to me about work today. Although I've publicly stated that I'm unavailable for work, it's nice to know I'm still in demand. This boosts the ego and might benefit the bank balance, as money may run out soon.

Another aspect that has changed since the operation is my approach to eating. I have almost dreaded my evening meal for the last few nights. I've been in real pain when going to bed. We're having a vegetarian, gluten-free carbonara pasta tonight, and for the first time, I'm going to bed without experiencing any pain this evening.

It could be due to having mint tea before bed, or perhaps things are improving. I may never know, but I've discovered that enjoying mint tea before bed is quite pleasant. I aim for an early night, hoping it prepares me for tomorrow when I return to the hospital.

21 January 2025

Another day and another hospital visit. Today, I hope to have the drain hanging from my tummy onto my leg removed. It's still giving out liquid this morning. It dropped from 200 mil yesterday to about 85 mil this morning, so I'm hopeful they might remove it.

I spend the morning before my hospital time catching up with colleagues from work, just trying to sort things out for my return. I really hope they remove this drain today, and then perhaps I can start making phone calls tomorrow about beginning some light work next week, mainly because I've discovered that I can't sit at my desk with this drain in me.

I arrive at the hospital at 11 am as planned, and today, I only have to wait for a relatively short time of 40 minutes.

When I see Sara, I mention that approx 110 mil came out of the drain, and she says I need to keep it in. I realise this process is a series of peaks and troughs, but this disappoints me deeply.

I can't stand up straight. I can't get comfortable, and I don't want this drain inside me any more, but I also accept that it's for the best.

They also need to run some tests. I'm told not to worry about them, but I'm also informed that there's a small chance they may have inadvertently damaged my insides during the surgery, so they need to test me while I'm there. Grrr, not what I wanted.

In the meantime, I have my wound redressed so that the waterproof component of the drain is nice and fresh because I noticed it peeling off. I resealed it myself with some surgical tape Emma gave me on Saturday.

I spend five minutes waiting for someone to redress my wound, and I feel disappointed. I'm upset and slightly scared, but that's all I allow myself to feel. There's no point in being upset or frightened beyond those five minutes. They'll tell me what's wrong, and then we'll figure out how to resolve it.

I provide a urine sample so they can check if they have cut me, and then I'll head home. I'll return in 72 hours.

Typically, the bag becomes more uncomfortable in the afternoon and evening. I literally can't find a comfortable position. I can't get the pipe to settle in a spot that isn't poking my freshly cut stomach, which is irritating. However, I also have to remember that this is just for 72 hours, and hopefully, when this comes off, I can begin the road to recovery.

This is a journey of peaks and troughs.

22 January 2025

Today is the first day Emma has returned to work since my surgery. She leaves the house at 7 am, and I feel really bad for her because, before all of that, she needs to walk the dogs, make me a drink and get me ready for the day. It's unfair on her, and I feel utterly useless.

Once Emma leaves, I sit in bed and watch YouTube. I've let the dogs come in since I'm staying in the spare room, hoping they won't jump on my stomach at night. Being awake means allowing them to lie beside me, and I love it.

I wish to begin working by 8 am.

I begin browsing my social media, hoping to find something I can engage with, searching for an opportunity to be productive. I end up making several phone calls to a few contacts regarding potential work in the future.

As part of my work, I deliver public speaking engagements at conferences and events. Before my operation, I took the time to inform the organisers of several events about my illness, expressing my hope to return in time to speak, but also acknowledging that I might not make it.

This morning, I find myself browsing the websites of some of the events where I'm scheduled to speak throughout this calendar year, and I notice that my name is no longer listed as one of the speakers on more than one occasion. Seeing this amplifies my mental anguish alongside my physical pain. A part of me thinks, "How dare they exclude me without consulting me first?"

However, I understand that in reality, these event organisers must consider the needs of those who pay to attend their events. They're ensuring the right level of insurance by removing my name and substituting it with incredible speakers.

It's something that I appreciate has to happen.

Still, I think, "I'll see you on a stage in the future and deliver a keynote that people will always remember."

You see, that's the **real** me. I'm self-centred. It's one of the things I intensely **dislike** about myself, but it also gives me confidence.

This confidence allows me to set my mind to something and achieve it; it helps manage my imposter syndrome, but keeping that confidence in check can be challenging for me on a daily basis.

I often have to remind myself of the need to balance this confidence and self-centredness with my ability because, frankly, my ability has never been as good as I hope it is.

I spend the rest of the day lying in my pain pit and sulking.

Emma returns from work at 6:30 pm, and I feel sorry for her again. She has been out of the house for nearly 12 hours and needs to walk the dogs right away, then cook for both of us because I can't even lift a saucepan.

Honestly, I feel terrible.

I'm in pain. The drain attached to my belly is driving me crazy, and I can't wait to have it removed.

On that note, the hospital calls me today. They inform me that my tests from yesterday were all good and they can remove the bag and the drain on Friday.

Woo hoo, I can't wait.

23 January 2025

Emma goes to work today at 7 am, just like she did yesterday, and I feel just as bad while Emma takes care of all the morning chores and walks the dogs.

Once again, I lie in bed and watch TV, bored out of my mind by 8 am. I used this quote today in a WhatsApp message to someone.

"My mind is writing cheques that my body cannot cash"

What I mean by that is simple: I want to get up. I want to go out, go for a run and sit at my desk. I want to be productive, yet all I can manage is working on getting out of bed, which takes me four minutes, showering with one arm and trying to cover up my bag.

Additionally, the fact that I've noticed my removal from the speakers list at certain events still weighs on my mind. I question whether I'm being unreasonable by admitting that it frustrates me. I understand that the world must go on even if I'm unwell, but it has genuinely bothered me.

Just as I'm thinking, "No, don't get angry," I receive an email from a large mailing list asking volunteers to do something that I had been individually asked to do in December 2024.

A large company asked me to do this, and I wanted to, but I decided it was best to inform them that I couldn't commit in January due to my surgery. However, if we could move it to February or March, there was a chance I could.

I opened up to them about something that had weighed on my mind for a long time, something I had carefully considered and reflected upon. I poured my thoughts and feelings into that conversation, hoping for understanding or at least a response. However, I was met with silence. It was incredibly hurtful to share such a personal part of myself and receive no acknowledgment in return. This lack of response made me feel dismissed and unimportant, as if my feelings didn't matter. It left me feeling vulnerable and rejected, amplifying the pain of not being heard or validated. I had hoped for a connection, but instead, I felt more alone than ever before.

Now I see them petitioning a mailing list, asking others to do it. I won't lie; it pisses me off that this reveals how expendable we all are and how we don't matter to anyone else. Yes, I'm writing this on the same day, so my emotions are high. But if this feeling remains when I publish this diary, it'll mean I've reviewed it and still feel the same way. (Edit – I still feel the same way).

So, my message to you, the reader, is that while people can tell you they care and support you, they'll truly mean it in that moment. However, the world moves on at a rapid pace, with or without you.

In moments like this, when you feel 10% of your usual self, an email like this one can destroy you momentarily. This is how I feel today.

I'm utterly destroyed, stripped of my confidence and marginalised.

All I really want is a hug; today, I cry a little.

24 January 2025

Today was a good day. It was the day that I finally had my bile bag removed. I want to dedicate this diary entry to a medical practitioner named Sara.

Top of Form

Bottom of Form

Firstly, Sara, thank you for acknowledging that removing my bile bag would be anything but slightly painful; that's somewhat of an understatement.

"I can't describe how this will feel."

These were Sara's words; her rationale was that she isn't male and has never experienced this herself.

It wasn't painful; it felt more like an electric shock coursing through my groin and radiating throughout my body. I described it as being kicked in the balls while tightly squeezing them; I apologise for being so graphic. That's exactly how it felt.

I believe that's the first time during this treatment that I'd made a noise and winced audibly. I really hope I don't have to experience that again any time soon.

To leave the hospital after my operation, I negotiated that I could go with the bag I mentioned, as long as I was willing to change it and return to the hospital to have it checked. Sara, the medical practitioner, recognised that I needed to sleep and rest much more than I needed hospital care, and she has been absolutely amazing throughout this journey.

Today, as she removed my bio bag, we engaged in an extensive conversation. We discussed the operation, my recovery, and my approach to healing. Additionally, we talked about the politics and logistics of having patients in a hospital, along with the challenges involved during their discharge. It can be particularly difficult for medical practitioners like Sara, as they have a duty of care to their patients, and some patients lack both the means and the desire to leave the hospital. Here I was, 11 days later, yet some individuals I had shared a ward with were still there today, due to a mixture of circumstances.

We talked about my case and my approach to it, and Sara said that I'm incredibly positive and that she supported these diary entries because she hopes that people get to read about the real experiences of cancer and not just the negative experiences.

So let me be real, Sara, if you're reading this – you're amazing. Your teams are incredible, and I just wanted to thank you for your care and your words of wisdom during this process. I also wanted to thank you for agreeing to my final question as I left your room today.

The question was simple: "Can I have a pint tonight?"

Her answer was, "Yes. You're well on your way to recovery and can do anything in moderation."

Thank you, Sara!

25 January 2025

It's a Saturday, and it's the first Saturday in several weeks that I haven't been preoccupied with thoughts of the upcoming operation or overly concerned about cancer.

There's not much to write about today. It's just a normal Saturday filled with relaxation, a good breakfast and watching my team, Liverpool FC, defeat Ipswich 4-1.

The Substack on which these diary entries are based now has over 70 subscribers; to me, this is madness, but it's wonderful to hear from people who find my words helpful on their journeys.

By 5 pm, the relaxing day has turned into a bit of energy, so I pop out to our local pub and have a couple of pints. It's so nice to enter the real world, and in this real world, we see someone who knows what's been going on, and they're pleased to see me at the bar. It's nice to know that people care. It's nice to know that people notice you when you're not there and are delighted when you return.

Thanks, Steven.

26 January 2025

Last night, I enjoyed eight and a half hours of sleep. Now that the bag is gone, my sleep has improved tremendously, and I can feel my recovery taking shape.

I also woke up this morning needing to change the dressing on my largest wound. I now realise that I have five distinct cuts on my stomach: two fairly small ones, one in my belly button, one next to it that's quite long, and the one that had the bile bag attached to it, which is still healing. I thought changing my dressing would gross me out, but it wasn't as bad as I thought.

I believe there's a takeaway from this entire diary and treatment: your mind can convince you that things will be awful. You can start to believe that things will be terrible, and therefore they seem that way. However, you can also find balance and recognise that while they may not be pleasant, you can overcome them, rise to the challenge, and help yourself by staying positive.

For me, that's my mantra during this treatment. These hurdles are just obstacles; you can jump over them, run through them, or even cheat and run around them.

The point is that you need to bypass them and get to the next hurdle, and that really is just life, as well as cancer treatment.

You may remember my trip to the middle-class farmers' market near my home just before Christmas, where I spent £14 on olives and onions. That market reopened today, but it's a bit further away, making the walk there and back a bit challenging.

Emma and I left home at 10 am and went to the market. This time, I spent only £8 and walked 3.5 km.

To provide some perspective, I walked 0.6 km last Monday and found it difficult. Walking nearly seven times that distance today and still finding it challenging yet achievable felt fantastic.

The rest of the day was spent patting myself on the back and looking at ultra runs in 2026.

27 January 2025

Today, I wake up feeling full of energy. I think it's the first day I've truly 'attempted' to spring out of bed since the operation. When I say 'attempted,' it's because I'm still in pain, so moving like I used to, just two weeks and one day ago, remains difficult.

But today feels like a good day. I have energy and am eager to return to work, so I call my clients to let them know I'm back and ready to go when they need me. It's lovely to hear them ask how I am and show interest in me; equally, it's delightful for me to be interested in them and hear how things have been going over the past few weeks. I'm not planning on diving in headfirst and working five days a week, but working some hours is better than working no hours. It'll keep my mind occupied and help me use this energy I can't harness for the next four to five weeks.

Today is also the first time I'll sit at my desk for any length of time. While I'm there, I receive an email stating that I've been voted one of the top 25 leaders in my professional field. My industry has approximately 10,000 people working in it, so being among that global top 25 makes me proud. I made the list last year, but this year, due to the cancer, I completely forgot that it could even be a possibility. Thus, receiving that email informing me that I've been nominated and named one of the top 25 fills me with immense pride.

However, I've lost sight of the importance of what I do over the past few weeks because, honestly, it doesn't seem as significant as fighting cancer. It doesn't feel as crucial as writing this diary, hoping someone will read it and find it helpful.

I have another interesting conversation today with a professional acquaintance who has lymphoma, a distinct type of cancer that affects the blood.

His condition is incurable, and he is struggling with the same demons that I contend with regarding positivity and negativity, fluctuating between highs and lows, looking at Google and worrying about what it reveals.

However, over half an hour, we engage in a meaningful conversation, exchanging thoughts on the indignity of having cancer and the accompanying pain at times. We also explore how it has provided us with a new perspective on life and how, in the midst of all the negativity, we stay positive and focused on looking ahead – not too far into the future, but far enough to make meaningful plans, enjoy our lives, and envision a future that isn't solely defined by cancer.

A future that isn't governed by cancer.

THE PHONE CALL

28 January 2025

28 January is my father's birthday, so I start the day by messaging him to wish him a happy birthday. Little do I know that I'll call him later with other news.

I also wake up to a message in my inbox today from Marie. Marie runs a community called Behind The Mask, which aims to help professionals in any sector remove the masks that we all wear to protect ourselves and others. It provides a space where we can discuss the truth about our real feelings and what we need to help us get by every day.

She plans to publish an extract from these diaries on their website.

- *https://www.linkedin.com/company/behind-the-mask-community.*

Engaging in that conversation is a wonderful way to begin the day, and I'm delighted that people are embracing these diary entries and deciding to share them with their audiences so that others can gain from them.

Today, I plan to support Emma as she goes to the hospital at London Bridge. Emma faces health challenges that could fill an entire collection of diaries. I plan to have a little mooch around Borough Market, perhaps buy myself something nice to eat, and then meet Emma after her appointment to visit a museum.

The phone call

We might even grab a drink and a bite to eat afterwards.

As we roll into London Bridge, my phone rings, and it's an unknown number. I answer, discovering that it's my surgeon's secretary. She explains that she'd like to book me in for an appointment this Thursday at 3:45 pm. I reply that I can't make it as Emma will be at work, suggesting that we could sort out another day.

Her reply is:

"I suggest you come on this day; it's something you need to do."

I take a breath and reply, "That sounds worrying. Should I be concerned?" I get little context at the end of the line, just to say it's probably best if I come in, and so, reluctant and worried, I accept the appointment.

Emma and I get off the train, both in a daze; the nice day out we had planned, our first since New Year, has just vanished into thin air. Emma begs me to join her for her appointment, mainly so I can get out, get some air and be occupied but the last thing I want is to sit in the hospital, so I walk into Borough Market, just walking, not looking at anything.

Now, to understand me, you need to know that I would normally buy a coffee and some cakes, explore all the other different foods, likely visit some clothing shops, and unnecessarily spend money. However, today I wander around aimlessly, not even paying attention to what's around me.

It's then that an idea strikes me. What if I call the nurses at my local Macmillan, who were also part of the multidisciplinary team meeting that discussed my case this morning, and ask them if they can share anything? The only problem is that I don't have their number, but thinking on my feet, I look back through these very diary entries and recall the day I called them to get my first set of results. I scroll back through my phone to that day and see that at 12:28 pm, I made the phone call that informed me the tumour was cancer.

For your information, it's probably worth having an overview of an MDT – multidisciplinary team.

- *https://www.bowelcanceruk.org.uk/about-bowel-cancer/treatment/*.

I call the number and explain the conversation I've just had. I mention that I'm tough enough to take bad news any time, but what I'm *not* is patient. I would appreciate knowing what's going on before Thursday if possible. The nurse, as always, is wonderful. She says she'll need to consult with her colleagues and call me back.

Emma and I meet after her appointment and head home. There are no shops, no lunch, no museum, and barely any conversation between us. The silence magnifies my anxiety and worry, as although I've been recovering well from the surgery I've received very little good news regarding this cancer so far.

This feels like I'm back on that Sunday night, on 1 December, when I first saw that tumour...

When we return home, I still haven't heard anything from the nurses, and my head's spinning. I don't know what to do. I'm desperate to call them back, but I don't want to be a burden.

After three hours, I decide to call them back, and when I do, I'm so glad I did. I speak to a lady named Jonna, and she tells me what they've found, so here goes.

During my operation, 19 lymph nodes were removed, and three of those tested positive for cancerous cells. This indicates that my cancer is classified as stage three, which also suggests that I should meet with an oncologist to discuss chemotherapy as the next step.

I'm sure there's more detail that the surgeon needs to share on Thursday, but by the end of the conversation, I feel much happier knowing what's coming next. I'm content that on Thursday, I'll learn more about my physical recovery from the surgery, and I've arranged my meeting with the oncologist for 11 February to discuss chemotherapy.

Readers of this book will notice that I'm doing my best to maintain a positive attitude throughout this journey. However, I've hinted at it before, but I'm vain.

I've reached the ripe age of 47 with a full head of dark hair and, if I may say so, a glorious beard. My biggest fear among all of this is losing that hair and that beard, which define me physically.

They're my comfort blanket, reassuring me that I'm here, confident, and ready to speak in front of you.

Imagining their disappearance frightens me greatly. But what's the alternative?

The alternative is to turn down chemotherapy, which would increase my risk of this cancer recurring. That would be a foolish move. Within an hour, I've gone from my head spinning to being fully focused on the next stage of this journey. Right now, I must continue to focus on my physical recovery. Then, in a few weeks, I will get to focus on chemotherapy and the joy that it's going to bring to my life.

STRESS, STRESS, STRESS

29 January 2025

Yesterday was a tough experience. I feel like I'm coping with the news of the chemotherapy much worse than I did with the news of the surgery.

I'll explain why this is.

Simply put, I want to reiterate what I said yesterday: I'm vain. I've come this far with a full head of hair and a beard, which I feel identify me as 'me'. I know I've mentioned this before, but I truly feel that way.

Last night, I spent too much time looking at the stories of other chemo patients and clinging to the terminology used to describe my cancer.

Those terms indicated 'Stage three' out of four stages. This frightens me immensely; however, I must realise that, technically speaking, I'm cancer-free.

Cancer has been removed from my body, and this chemotherapy is there to mop up any remaining cells. It's like an insurance policy, so to speak. Like any insurance, it'll cost me. There's a trade-off, which might include my hair and beard. It could also be fatigue or pins and needles, but this time next year, I hope it'll all be over.

I was scheduled to return to work with my client today, and after much consideration, I decide it was the right decision. Working today means that I can be fully prepared to resume work next week, as I feel that I've physically recovered quite well from the surgery. I just hope the surgeon agrees with my assessment when I see him tomorrow.

One thing I suffered from last night was the quality of my sleep. I tossed and turned, worrying and thinking too much about chemotherapy. Still, if I may be so crude, I also had a stomach ache because yesterday I told Emma, "Blow it, put some chilli in the rice, and let's have some broccoli." That introduction of fibre is something my stomach isn't used to.

I'll spare you any more details. Needless to say, I woke up a few times during the night. I also woke up Norris, our dog, who has chosen to start sleeping with me. Now I need to consider when I can return to our marital bedroom because sleeping alone is not what I signed up for.

My day at work is quite good. It's nice to talk to people again. It's great to engage my mind in topics not centred around cancer. I also receive phone calls from friends who matter – individuals who understand me and know what I'm going through.

On a scale of one to ten, it's probably a 'seven' day, and I'm recording this pre-game. Still, Liverpool will play their final Champions League match against PSV Eindhoven tonight. The result doesn't matter because we've already qualified, so I might sit back, watch the night unfold, and see which of Liverpool's rivals fail to progress to the group stages.

I apologise to all non-football fans.

30 January 2025 – The surgeon

Last night wasn't my best night's sleep. I'm still really hung up on this stage three cancer diagnosis; in my mind, I completely understand that the tumour has been removed and that I'll be undergoing chemotherapy to reduce the chances of it returning. However, I feel more scared about today's meeting with the surgeon than I have about any of my meetings so far. I feel increasingly irrational, and I guess this is what anxiety feels like, which is something I'm now getting used to.

Today is really about talking with the surgeon, but fortunately, I have the wonderful distraction of chatting with my friend Lucy, who has co-authored a book with me. The book is called *Allyship Actually*, if you're interested.

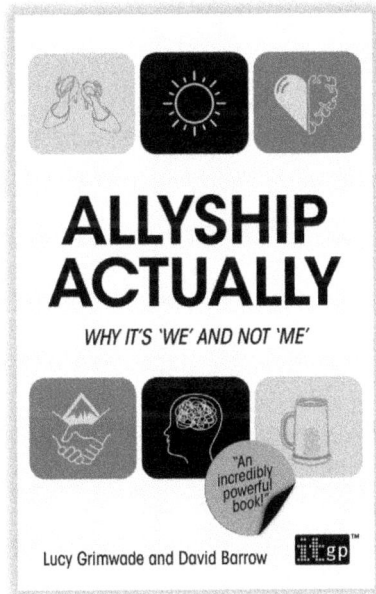

Allyship Actually **Cover**

Lucy and I talk extensively about our days and all our day-to-day happenings. We also discuss my situation.

Stress, stress, stress

I hope Lucy won't mind my saying that she has also struggled with anxiety in the past. She helps me compartmentalise my thoughts and begin to understand them. It's helpful that Lucy is a coach and can empathise.

Lucy, thank you so much for helping me out today. It means the world.

Emma and I head to the hospital at around midday. I spend the entire trip just wandering around in a daze.

When we arrive at the hospital, I can feel my heart pounding and my stress levels escalating; all of this feels insane as I'm fairly certain about what I'm going to be told:

"The cancer is gone, and the chemo is just to reduce recurrence."

We're called in to see the surgeon right on time, which is a relief!

Here are my stress levels before, during and after my consultation:

118

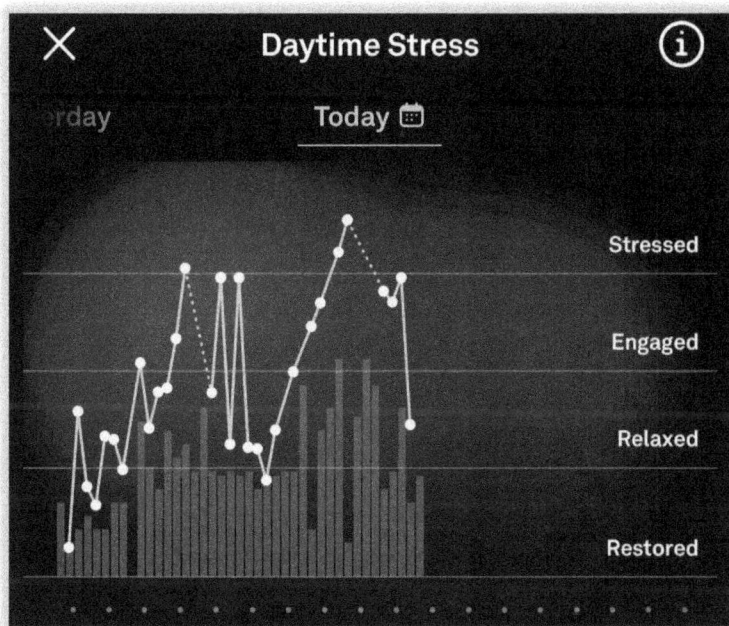

Stress Readings

What you see here are my stress readings from my Oura Ring. This ring monitors my health and is one of the reasons I visited the GP in the first place.

I've never felt as though I was suffering from anxiety before all of this, but I've now experienced it on multiple occasions, especially today in the moments leading up to seeing the surgeon; I've come to understand what 'scanxiety' means.

I don't know why, but I can't shake the feeling that there'll be bad news in this meeting. We enter the room, and like us, the surgeon wears his mask. He says we should remove ours, but he'll keep his on since he has a bit of a cold.

We discuss the surgery, and he explains that it went well and that they believe they got the vast majority, if not all, of the cancer.

The surgeon is surprised that I already know that 3 of my 19 lymph nodes contained cancerous cells and, therefore, I'll be recommended for chemotherapy. He states that it's the right thing to do, and the oncologist will provide more information about the side effects when we meet on 11 February.

He mentions from his experience that the combination of drugs used in this treatment does not result in hair loss. I hope he's right because it's something I'm afraid of. I also express my anxiety because my cancer has been referred to as stage three out of four; he nods and says it's normal – but this treatment is to mop up anything they may have missed; it's just a set of troops doing a sweep.

We discuss my wounds further. He inspects my stomach, indicating that I'm healing well.

I had a wound that's still covered, which is where my drain was until last week. He peels back the plaster and says, "Wow, that's amazing, we can just leave that off."

So that's it. I no longer have any plasters or dressings on my stomach. He explains that the pain I'm experiencing is completely normal, and I'm managing it well.

Before we depart, he shares one last comment. "If you want one, you should go and have a glass of wine or two this evening."

I ask if I can have a Guinness. "Good man," he retorts.

If you look at that picture of my Oura Ring, you can see how I shift from stressed to relaxed in an instant; that's thanks to him. I never thought I was someone who looked up to authority, but I'm someone who recognises expertise.

He discussed my cancer, allowed us to engage in conversation, and explained things in a manner that inspired my trust. Rightly or wrongly, that trust made me feel relaxed.

Thanks, Mr Shihab.

Emma mentions that she could see the stress visibly leave me during our conversation. I feel so relieved to leave the hospital.

I'm still worried, I'm still concerned, I'm still absolutely fucking petrified of chemotherapy, but I'm ready to start preparing to take it on. Whatever it gives me, I'll fight back; however, it makes me feel, I'll try to be positive, and hopefully this time in six months when I see the doctor again, I'll be cancer-free. Let's see how we go.

31 January 2025

My day begins shortly after midnight. I went to bed at around 10:10 pm after Emma and I had had a couple of drinks, then decided to order curry. When I spoke to the surgeon yesterday, I asked if I could reintroduce normal food, including vegetables and fruit. He said absolutely.

In his words, "What's the worst that could happen? Diarrhoea."

It might be too much information, but he wasn't far off. I woke up just after 12 am, feeling a little gurgled, shall we say? I went to the loo and realised I should be sitting down rather than standing up. I'll leave you with that lovely image, but it kept me busy until about half two in the morning.

At least I was awake and laughing.

When I finally get out of bed later, there isn't much for everyone to do, so we choose to relax. Emma is supposed to meet a friend in Clapham, but the weather is awful, and my mood is still a little dark. I still can't quite get over this chemo thing; it's strange. I know I'm being unreasonable, but sometimes the mind plays tricks on us.

In the middle of the afternoon, the hospital calls me to ensure I'm fully aware that I'll be going for chemotherapy. I explain that I am, but one thing I forgot to do yesterday was ask the doctor for my grading and staging of my cancer.

It's been classified as T3N1M0.

Now, for those of you who don't have cancer, you might be wondering what I'm talking about, so let me break it down:

- T3 means the cancer has penetrated quite a way through my bowel, but not entirely.
- N1 means that the cancer has spread to three nearby lymph nodes; I understand that this can be two to three, not just three.
- M0 indicates that the cancer has not metastasised anywhere else in my body. We knew this prior to the operation, as I had CT scans and MRI scans, but it's still good to affirm.

This, however, is the root of my anxiety: what if it spreads? What if it's already spreading? These thoughts aren't sensible, but they keep crossing my mind.

We nip out to our local town to buy groceries and then stay home. We watch TV, eat junk food all day, and relax. Both of us are in bed by 9 pm and asleep by 9:05 pm.

By the end of the day, I have settled my anxiety around chemotherapy, and the longest, most depressing month of the year is over.

Thank fuck for that.

1 February 2025

The longest month of the year is finally over. Back on 31 December, I hoped that my new year would start on 1 February, which is the mindset I've woken up with today. I'm still feeling out of sorts when it comes to dealing with chemotherapy, but I think I've wrapped my head around the fact that technically, I no longer have cancer. This chemotherapy is intended to reduce the chances of it returning. I feel better about this when I think of it as a few soldiers entering my body to mop up whatever may be left of the cancer.

Emma and I should be at a friend's 40th birthday party today, but the celebration is 240 miles away. Back in December, I informed them that we couldn't attend. That was the right decision, even though I feel much better than three weeks ago. I'm still not fully recovered and couldn't sit in a car for four hours. Additionally, I wouldn't do myself any favours by going to a party and getting drunk.

So instead, today, we take it easy for the first part of the day. I do some work and prepare myself to start working fully next week. I research chemotherapy-related diets and talk with my good friends Tim and his wife, Shona, about what's happening in their lives and their new home. They have also faced a struggle with cancer in the past, so being able to converse with them and understand their experiences is incredibly helpful. I want to express my gratitude to them;

if you're reading this, thank you so much for everything you've done for me.

This afternoon, I again have two screens running: one to watch Dorking in their football game and the other to view Liverpool, who lead 2-0 away from home against Bournemouth. This means we're still on top of the league, which distracts me from this cancer.

Later in the afternoon, we meet our friend Doug at the local pub to watch the rugby. England loses the game, but in fairness, we don't really pay much attention to it. We're busy catching up and chatting. I don't drink a lot, at least not for me, but it's all good. It's such a lovely day; we get to pretend this horrible thing isn't happening.

All that said, I'm knackered. It's amazing how a bit of socialising can get to me, and I'm in bed by 9 pm, ready for a good sleep. I'm hoping to move back to our marital bed tomorrow, as so far, I've been staying in my own room to ensure that one of our dogs doesn't jump on me during the night.

Maybe tomorrow, I'll move back in.

2 February 2025

Emma and I go to the gym for the second time in two days this morning. This time, I set the machine to 5.5 km per hour with an incline of 1, which is a little faster than the other day. With the added incline, frankly, I'm bored, but I know it's really good for me to get out and do a bit of exercise, as I'm finding it difficult to muster the enthusiasm to go for a walk around the block.

But it's nice to exercise, and then we can nip out to get a coffee on this lovely, sunny, frosty winter morning.

While poor Emma takes both dogs out, I sit back, relax and listen to a record my brother-in-law bought me. This kind of thing helps me unwind, and I enjoy it a lot, which is why I'm sitting there. However, I begin thinking about my nutrition. I want to ensure that I'm as healthy as possible during chemotherapy. I recognise the impact on my immunity, so I want to ensure that what I eat is genuinely beneficial.

I contact the Macmillan group on their chat line and speak to a lovely lady named Pauline, who gives me some great advice and sends me some awesome information about increasing my fibre intake, as well as getting counselling for a part of my journey that I'm really struggling with during chemotherapy. I've never considered counselling before, but I think it'll be helpful in this case, and I would also like to explore it because, in the last week, I've signed up for a master's programme in psychology, counselling and coaching, as I'm really interested in how the brain works. During this time, I've discovered how powerful it can be, both positively and negatively.

After discussing nutrition in this entry, I quickly disregard it. We receive a message from our neighbours asking if we'd like to go out for a pint later, and I say yes, which shows I can't be that interested in nutrition. However, I also think I should take advantage of these opportunities. It's not like we're going to go crazy, and we'll eat plenty of veggies later, so we'll see how that affects our fibre intake.

I feel today that the weather is making a massive difference to my approach; just having a bit of brightness and sunshine feels so good. I truly hope that during this chemotherapy stage, I'm allowed to go on holiday to a place where I can soak up some sunshine and warmth, as I really need it right now. I've always suffered in winter with seasonal affective disorder (SAD), but I'm really feeling it now. It would be great to get out, enjoy some sun and just relax for a bit.

Today, I also receive a wonderful review for the book I wrote with Lucy. It's so lovely to read. It's the little things like this that are so helpful in recovery, keeping your mind positive and alert. Thank you, Mo; I really appreciate that.

3 February 2025

As you know, I write these diaries entries each day, and I don't expect this will be a long entry, but let's see how it goes.

Today marks the beginning of my first real working week since the surgery. My goal this week is to avoid the word I'm about to say: cancer. I have no medical appointments scheduled, so I can focus on living a relatively normal life.

Or so I think. Halfway through the day, I get a text from my GP surgery saying they've arranged a telephone appointment for me at 5 pm today to speak to a cancer nurse. I don't even know what they want to talk to me about.

The working day serves as a lovely distraction; it's nice to catch up with people, understand what's happening, and begin contributing to the world in a way that isn't limited to just giving blood or getting my temperature checked. It's a good day – not much to write home about, really.

The nurse calls me at 5:20 pm, and it turns out to be a lovely chat. She reassures me that she is there to support me and asks how I'm doing. We share a laugh about my bowel movements, which are actually quite good. She helps ease my mind about the upcoming chemotherapy, and bless her, she tells me that her own husband recently received a cancer diagnosis and underwent an operation last week. We both chuckle about how neither her husband nor I can walk our large dogs, and how challenging it is for the spectators – in this case, her and my wife – who have to watch someone go through this while also providing support, both physically and mentally. It truly isn't a small thing, and I genuinely appreciate everything Emma does for me.

For those supporting someone on a cancer journey, you may find this useful:

- *https://www.bowelcanceruk.org.uk/about-bowel-cancer/living-with-and-beyond-bowel-cancer/emotional-wellbeing/supporting-someone-with-bowel-cancer/*.

Today is also the first night I'm going to sleep in our marital bed. I feel like I'm recovering well enough to manage the dogs potentially jumping on me, and it's lovely to return to my own bed. Yes, the dogs do jump up on the bed, but they're considerate enough not to jump directly on me.

Poor Emma has to contort herself around them during the night. Isn't it wonderful to get back to normal?

4 February 2025

Today is World Cancer Day. It's a day that I never even knew existed until last week.

Currently, these diaries about my cancer journey are shared on my LinkedIn. I've been very open there about what I'm experiencing because I believe prospective clients should be aware. I also think that if people stop reaching out, then I don't want to maintain connections with them anyway.

I've also had my story featured in a LinkedIn community called Behind The Mask after they reached out to me. Their aim is to help people drop the masks we all wear, revealing our insecurities and worries.. They encourage us to be more open and vulnerable, and I think it's a great cause.

I've spent most of my corporate career pretending to be something I'm not. I've always tried to be my authentic self, but probably only 70% of it. When I share my story, I'm not looking for pity. Honestly, the point of this diary and sharing my experiences is to hopefully help someone in the future get checked early enough, so they don't find themselves like me, dealing with stage three cancer. If that happens, I will be over the moon.

I return to the gym this morning, walking on the machine when I see Wendy, the receptionist from the hospital's colonoscopy department. She looks slightly surprised to see me at the gym, but I reassure her that I'm just walking. I manage to cover 3.3 km in 30 minutes. I'm on the verge of running three weeks too early, which makes me think about that half-marathon I mentioned earlier in the diary. Could I do it? I believe I could, but I really need to see what happens at the chemotherapy appointment on 11 February before I commit to that. Overall, I'm feeling good today, and I hope that continues for a long time.

In recognition of World Cancer Day, I've come across many posts, both positive and negative. I've decided to find purpose as a bowel cancer patient. This begins with my intention to form a community or self-help group. I'm not certain if I'll proceed, but if I do, I'd like to use BOWEL as its acronym. This is what I've come up with.

I have no idea if this will lead anywhere, but if you believe a community could assist, please let me know through my email at the back of this book.

- **Bringing:** Providing active engagement and community stories
- **Optimism:** Aiming for a positive, hopeful approach to facing cancer
- **Wellness:** Focusing on holistic health and being in charge of your recovery
- **Enablement:** Independence to take charge and not be defined by the big 'C'
- **Light:** Represent hope, healing and guidance through difficult times

And just as I settle down for the day with a peaceful mind, I get a huge slap in the face.

At 5:15 pm, I receive an online letter inviting me to a telephone appointment tomorrow at 2:30 pm. This is for a follow-up on my colorectal surgery, which immediately triggers an intense wave of anxiety and worry.

The suddenness and late notice of this request leave me feeling disoriented as if I have been abruptly pulled from a delicate balance into chaos. My mind races with questions and uncertainties, each one a cruel exposure of my vulnerability – a vulnerability I try to hide behind a mask of positivity.

I feel angry and frustrated, battling a sense of helplessness that only intensifies my anxiety. It's challenging not to dwell on the unknowns accompanying medical follow-up visits; they're more than just routine check-ins. Each appointment can feel like a checkpoint in a very difficult journey, reminding me of the fragility of my health and mind.

The mere thought of discussing my health again weighs heavily on me. It transforms my evening into a looming confrontation with my fears. It feels as if I'm trapped in a cycle of unease, where each appointment brings a flood of emotions – fear of the unknown and worry about the future, overshadowing any fleeting moments of hope or relief I may have felt.

At this moment, I feel powerless, struggling to regain a sense of control over my circumstances. Poor Emma tries to help me rationalise, but I feel like I'm losing it. Even I know I'm doing it, but I can't control it – I feel as if this is the closest I've ever come to a panic attack.

5 February 2025

Last night, I managed to regain some of the controllable aspects of my life.

It began with a call to my GP; I thought the lady I spoke to on Monday might be able to help me, but it turned out she wasn't there.

However, I was able to speak with her receptionist, who informed me that I hadn't been sent for any referrals, suggesting that I wasn't scheduled for a scan or a blood test.

After that, I called Macmillan. They explained that these situations weren't unusual, albeit poorly timed, which gave me a sense of control and allowed me to sleep.

This morning, I began work and decided to set aside everything until the call at 4:30 pm. To my surprise, I received a call from the hospital at 9:30 am. They informed me that I would be speaking with my Enhanced Recovery Nurse to check in and see how things were going.

I let out a sigh of relief upon hearing this.

Honestly, I recognise that my thoughts and feelings were quite irrational last night. Since November, I haven't received a single call to deliver encouraging news or even to inform me that my situation has remained unchanged.

My mind tends to gravitate toward analysis, and with a lack of communication, I found myself spiralling into anxious thoughts. The only scenario I could imagine was that the multidisciplinary team convened on Tuesday and must have come across some devastating news that they were withholding from me. I'm fully aware that such thoughts are not grounded in reality; they're a product of my fears. However, it's challenging to maintain rational thinking when grappling with the overwhelming presence of cancer in your life. This emotional turmoil is a natural response to the uncertainty that cancer patients often face, taking a toll on both the mind and spirit. We crave information and clarity, yet the absence of communication can leave us feeling isolated and fearful, amplifying our worries and uncertainties.

As it turns out, my meeting at 2:30 pm went well. They're very happy with my progress and are pleased to let me move on and speak to the oncologist next Tuesday to learn more about chemotherapy. Funnily enough, I still don't have an official appointment for Tuesday, even though they tell me its happening.

This is not something I allow myself to be concerned with this evening; I eat and head to bed early to recover.

6 February 2025

Today was a good day. I wasn't thinking about cancer; I was able to do some work for my own business and for the book I've recently released with Lucy (*Allyship Actually*).

Before we caught up, I had Emma drop me off in our local town. I grabbed a coffee, did some shopping, and walked home over some steep hills. Halfway up one of those hills, I realised I wasn't as fit as I used to be.

Lucy and I met at 11 am, and we had a good chat. Later, we met with an organisation that we'll be presenting to in a few weeks. It was just a nice, normal day – nothing to write about, but these ordinary days are actually something to write about at this moment.

I'm sorry to the non-football fans and Tottenham fans out there because Liverpool beat Tottenham 4-0 in the second leg of the semi-final tonight. They're on their way to Wembley.

Nice one, Redmen! You're keeping my spirits up this season.

7 February 2025

Another normal day – two in a row, wow!

I went to the gym and walked 3.5 km in 30 minutes. A week ago, it was only 2.75 km. I'm wondering if I'm starting to push myself too much.

Today, Lucy and I presented via Teams to a UK-based federation and the Women in Technology community. It was great to get back to what I love – speaking to people – and I hope we pass on the message that allyship should exist in this world.

At 2 pm, once this was done, I had a choice: stay at home or go out for a drink. So that's what I did! I went to the pub, had a bite to eat, chatted with friends, and was back home by 6 pm – happy and fulfilled.

A day when cancer didn't enter my thoughts.

8 February 2025

I'm sorry if the last two days of this diary haven't really aligned with what you're looking for. You're here to read about cancer, but from my perspective, you're actually reading about days when cancer isn't dominating my life.

And I'm here for it.

Today, our friends Denise and Tim came to meet us, along with their children, Oliver and Joseph. We hung out for the whole day, went out for a couple of drinks, had a really nice pub lunch, and then returned to our house to watch England in the Six Nations rugby, who surprisingly beat France in one of the best rugby games I've seen.

This morning was also the first time I joined Emma to walk the dogs in four weeks. Usually, this is my job, but Emma has been doing this brilliantly twice a day every day while I've been unable to. She still has two weeks to go, but I can now join her on the walk and help out.

9 February 2025

The worst thing about today was that Liverpool lost in the FA Cup to Plymouth. Usually, this would upset me, but today I have bigger things to worry about. Well done, Plymouth; it was well-deserved. You can't win them all, Liverpool.

A much more enjoyable aspect was that our friends Andrea and Tommy came to visit. They had wanted to come since my surgery but also wished to give me some space before arriving. It was nice to catch up, have a cup of tea, chat, and truly reconnect since we hadn't seen each other in a little while. I honestly believe they expected to see someone unwell, but they were pleasantly surprised to find me looking fairly normal – or as normal as I can appear. It was a lovely day, and that's about it; nothing more to say.

10 February 2025

Another working day has arrived, and having work, at least for now, is a great distraction for me. I only have this week left, and I intend to make the most of it. I also hope to take on extra work in the future weeks.

I can only wish for some extra work because tomorrow I'm meeting with the oncologist to discuss my chemotherapy. Honestly, I think I've mentioned this before: I've found the prospect of chemotherapy to be much more challenging than I ever found the thought of surgery. For me, surgery was a matter of me versus the pain; it was about excelling in recovery and trying to surpass the experiences of others that I've seen online.

Chemotherapy is different; I can't escape it, and I can't pretend it's not there. I have to confront it and deal with it. I think I'm just about ready to accept that I'll have to endure something I would never wish on anyone for the next three to six months. But without it, all I'm doing is giving cancer the best chance to return and forcing me to go through all this again.

So swallow it up, Buttercup; my new dawn of normality must fade as I prepare to come to terms with chemotherapy.

11 February 2025

Thankfully, my oncology appointment today is at 9:20 am, which means no waiting around or feeling anxious. I can wake up, go to the gym, use that machine, and walk for 3.5 km. That half hour really clears my head, and in the meantime, Emma and I have compiled a list of questions we want to ask the oncologist.

We arrive at the hospital at 9:05 am and are immediately taken to a room where I'm weighed and measured for height. What's amusing about this is that they measure my height as almost two inches shorter than a month ago. I don't believe I've shrunk, and I'm wearing the same shoes.

I'm also not six feet tall like I was a month ago; today, I'm 5 feet 10, which really dents my confidence. However, I'lost weight post op but have gained some back in the weeks since, , which is a good thing because, frankly, I felt like I had lost too much post-op.

I really need to pay more attention to my diet.

I've been trying to reintroduce vegetables and fruits while cutting out biscuits, crisps, pasta and white bread. The problem is that I've started experiencing stomach pain as a result of eating healthier foods, making it easier to revert to my old habits. I really want to break out of that loop.

That said, I've been eating live yoghurt and drinking Actimel every day, along with vitamin D, slow-release vitamin C, magnesium, amino acids and iron. I must remember to ask the oncologist if I can continue to take these when I'm on treatment.

At 9:25 am, we sit down with the assistant oncologist – a really nice man – who takes me through their plans.

We're looking at three months of chemotherapy treatment. I'll need to have a PICC line, and I'll have to go to Guildford, which is about 45 minutes away, to receive my treatment once a month on a Friday.

So, at least that means my weekends are ruined from now until June. Once I have my infusion, I will spend two weeks taking tablets and have a week off before the cycle starts again.

If, like me, you have wondered what on earth a PICC line is, I hope this helps – it certainly helped me:

- *https://www.bowelcanceruk.org.uk/news-and-blogs/this-is-bowel-cancer-blog/take-your-picc/*.

With any luck, I'll be finished by June. The oncologist takes me through the list of side effects, which, frankly, is longer than my arm. The most likely side effects appear to be tingling fingers due to nerve damage; nausea; loss of appetite; and lethargy. Equally, I'm told that someone of my age and fitness could well sail through this. I'm not sure I'll sail through this, but if I get lucky, I'll be really happy.

I immediately ask him a simple yet important question: "Will I lose my hair?" His response delights me: "From one bearded man to another, it's unlikely; some patients see thinning, but hair loss is rare."

At that moment, I genuinely want to hug him and tell him what a handsome bastard he is – because he truly is. He resembles Liverpool goalkeeper Alisson Becker and is wearing nice shoes. In fact, I'm starting to wonder if I have a man crush.

I'm delighted that this will only be for three months. As a sports fan, I now view this as somewhat akin to a boxing camp. For those who may not know, boxers generally train rigorously for 12 weeks before any fight. That's 12 weeks when they put their lives on hold, 12 weeks focused on one goal and one outcome, and 12 weeks dedicated to setting themselves up for success. So, that's what I'm going to do; I'm going to set myself up for success.

I ask the oncologist many questions, and I'll list those below. One of them is whether I can continue taking my vitamins. He tells me that magnesium is really good in this scenario and that I should keep taking my vitamins outside of vitamins C and D.

I'm also allowed to exercise and have the occasional drink. Overall, it's not a bad result, although let's see how this diary unfolds in the coming weeks.

I apologise that today is a long entry, but I think this is one of the most important entries I'll make in the diary. Physically, I feel ready to do this, but we need to wait another three weeks, so it won't look like our start until 7 March. Mentally, I also feel in a good place to do this; knowing that it's three months and not six is really helpful. It gives me something to focus on, to think that maybe in June, I can start to put this behind me.

I have the chance to participate in a trial on developing a cancer vaccine. It simply requires my consent to allow some cells from my removed tumour to be collected, as well as a blood test. This blood test will check for the presence of what is referred to as cancer DNA, or ctDNA, in my system; reportedly, only 10% of people tested have it.

If I test positive, I'll be eligible for the trial, and if accepted, they'll develop a personalised vaccine for me. Perhaps more importantly, that research could lead to a vaccine for the general public. If I can help even one person in the future, as well as myself, then this will have all been worth it.

Enclosed below are the questions we asked the oncologist. I included these because if you're reading this and need to see an oncologist, I genuinely hope they're helpful.

The truth is, they answered the questions as they went along. I didn't ask many of these questions; I was just ticking them off as he spoke using the Notes app on my mobile phone.

However, having that in my head going in was incredibly useful, as it enabled me to focus on what he was saying rather than just listening and nodding. That approach might work for you, or it might not.

Either way, I hope you find these questions useful.

- *How long will the treatment take?* **A – 3 months.**
- *What form will it take?* **A – Intravenous via a PICC line and tablets.**
- *Where will it take place?* **A – Guildford and home.**
- *Is there a timetable?* **A – Guildford on a Friday, blood tests on the preceding Tuesday, and tablets at home.**

- *What are the known side effects and their probabilities?* A – A list as long as my arm, but mainly fizzy fingers, lethargy and loss of appetite.
- *I'm self-employed and speak publicly; is my appearance likely to change?* A – My hair may thin a little, but it should not be noticeable.
- *What does this do to the probability of recurrence?* A – It improves my chances of recurrence by 15%.
- *Can I run?* A –Yes!
- *Can I get focused nutritional advice?* A – No, I can get generic advice, but it's best to seek this specialist advice elsewhere.
- *Can I fly/go abroad?* A – It's best not to.
- *Can I drink alcohol?* A – In moderation.
- *Will my immune system be compromised?* A – Yes, quite a bit. I'll keep taking my supplements that help.

12 February 2025

Yesterday's consultation with the oncologist sent a wave of relief through me. Understanding how the treatment will be administered and where and when it'll happen is reassuring. It gives me another plan to focus on, so much so that I went to work today and barely thought about the cancer. The only thoughts I had were about my diet. I'm still struggling to incorporate fibre into my meals without it causing me pain or, dare I say, unpleasant gas. That's something I need to address, but other than that, it's a good day.

13 February 2025

Today, I spent the day researching nutrition. I asked a nurse a question about it during the oncology appointment, but I suspect they'll send me some literature that I've already read.

I started searching for nutritional advice and holistic approaches in areas specific to cancer and came across a place called Embracing Nutrition.

I sent them a note explaining my predicament, including how I'd like to maintain my strength and immune system while undergoing chemotherapy. It's important to me to regain some control and reduce potential side effects. Interestingly, I received a response from them that evening, and we're scheduled to chat next Tuesday.

This evening, Emma and I are going to the cinema to watch the new Bridget Jones film – our first 'date night' in quite some time. The film is OK, but even here in the darkness of a cinema, I end up overhearing one lady speaking to another about a colonoscopy that led to a cancer diagnosis. It's so hard to escape this bloody disease.

14 February 2025

It's Valentine's Day, so I woke Emma up with flowers this morning. It's reciprocal, as Emma shares some gifts with me; today probably stands out more than Emma's birthday.

After breakfast, we start to clean up the house because our good friends Daniel and Sam, along with their children Bradley and Betsy – who are also our godchildren – are coming to visit today. It'll be a fun weekend, and this will be the first time I've seen them since my diagnosis. I'm going to do my best not to get emotional.

The crew arrive late afternoon, and we catch up as we always do over a pint. It's a lovely afternoon and evening. We prepare some food for the kids and some for ourselves, then just sit and chat. Nothing major to write home about, but just another one of those moments when you forget that you've got cancer and that you have to go through three months of chemo.

15 and 16 February 2025

I've consolidated these two days together because they won't be what you, the reader, are here for; they're not about cancer.

They're great days – just us: Dan, Sam and the kids hanging out.

Bradley and I are playing FIFA, a game where I can just about keep up with him now, but at ten years old, he's likely to start beating me soon.

He and I are also playing Gran Turismo, a game I can still beat him at, which is good for me.

We just hang out, chat, eat and drink, and we've moved past the fact that I'm going through all this treatment. It's more about us enjoying a nice, wholesome weekend together. But for you, the reader, you might not really want to know about that, I guess. What you probably want to know is that there comes a point in this cancer journey where it starts to fade from your primary thoughts, where positive moments can overshadow it, where you can almost pretend it's not there. I hope I've reached that point, or at least a stage where I can distract myself long enough to feel good.

17 February 2025

Daniel, Samantha, Bradley and Betsy are leaving us today.

The last time they left, Betsy cried all the way home, but this time, she doesn't, which is a bit of a result.

It's so sad to see them go; the house feels so quiet, and I worry that I might crash back into reality. Yet, in truth, I don't.

I spend my time working and looking more into nutrition and holistic nutrition for when I'm going through the chemotherapy. I've discovered some really interesting things, so I'm quite looking forward to speaking with a nutritionist.

Other than that, it's a day of work, returning to the grind, and figuring out where my next job will come from. I've now got 13 days left. I'm unsure what we'll do for money once that time ends.

A couple of calls have come in with offers of potential work, and I find myself torn between letting them know I'm going through chemo or not. I decide to inform them. I'd much rather reach a point in this process where my chemo doesn't stop me from getting the work done later down the line. I prefer to be transparent, and frankly, if someone doesn't want to employ me because I have chemotherapy coming up, then I don't want to work with them.

Forget them; I'll move on to somewhere that values human kindness and my skills.

FIVE WEEKS DOWN, ONE TO GO (TILL I CAN GO FOR A RUN)

18 February 2025

Today is my first day at work. I'm in back-to-back meetings all day – on a typical day, this is not unusual.

Living in this cycle of meetings is something I dislike on a normal day; I'd probably say that I hate it. However, I love it today.

It's a huge distraction to move forward and feel like I'm truly accomplishing something that isn't centred around me and this dreadful cancer. I really enjoy it, but I also recognise that I have only 12 days left and still need to find a job.

Later in the day, I speak to Suzy from Embracing Nutrition, who will help me with my nutrition.

We're going to devise a plan that addresses the chemotherapy side effects and maybe even eliminates them.

I need a plan that gives me energy – one that will likely improve my diet because recently I've only been eating junk. I've been doing this because eating good food hurts, but I really need to overcome that and start getting nutrients back into my body.

I'm looking forward to this, and additionally, we're now less than a week away from when I can first go back for a run, and oddly, I'm feeling nervous about it since I still have slight pain; things still hurt and ache. I just have to get over it and see how it goes.

19 February 2025

Today is Wednesday, and in my new working life, it's my last day at work for the week. I'm now only working across three days most weeks, much of which is designed to help my recovery and also space out my engagement period with my current client – fantastic people who are so patient with me.

It's been a good day, made even better by my good friend Tim popping over to visit us for the night. We're also joined by Emma's parents, who are stopping by on their way to Scotland. It's great to catch up with them all.

Tim and his wife, Shona, have been rocks throughout this cancer experience. Unfortunately, they too have faced their own struggles with cancer, so having people to lean on, learn from and talk to is essential in this situation. My advice to anyone going through a tough time is to reach out to your friends because they're the ones who will truly support you.

If someone doesn't support you, they're not your friend.

Thank you, Tim. Thank you, Shona. And thank you to everyone who has supported me throughout this journey. As is the way with this diary, I watch Liverpool play tonight, and they draw 2-2 with Aston Villa. I wonder if that's a point dropped or a point gained.

20 February 2025

I'm now five weeks and three days post-surgery, and I was told that after six weeks, I can start to resume normal activities, but I cheat. I take both dogs out for a walk today, and it's lovely to walk them both. We don't do anything too hectic; they're not pulling me too much, but I can definitely feel their strength much more than I used to. I think it's just something I need to get used to, both physically and mentally. There's still that little worry in the back of my mind that I could hurt myself, but it goes fine.

Today, I manage to hopefully secure some work as an author and speaker, so all in all, a good day.

21 February 2025

Today is an interesting day.

When I saw the oncologist last week, I was asked if I'd be interested in participating in a cancer vaccine study. Essentially, the study aims to determine if I have cancerous DNA, also known as ctDNA, in my body; this helps researchers understand whether I'm among those individuals who are more predisposed to cancer than previously thought.

In my case, if the test is positive it would also indicate a higher likelihood of recurrence of my bowel cancer. If that's the case, I could potentially enter the study, where a vaccine will be developed to help prevent or reduce the chances of recurrence.

Additionally, this research will contribute to creating a vaccine for future cancer patients, which I'm enthusiastic about participating in.

What is ctDNA? ctDNA are small pieces of DNA found in the bloodstream when cancer cells die. Doctors take a sample of blood to look for ctDNA and to find specific changes (mutations) in the DNA.

Finding these changes may help to plan treatment. They may also help to assess how well treatment is working or to see if a cancer has come back.

As they describe on the Cancer Research UK website:

> *"A trial is looking at ctDNA in people with stage two or three colorectal cancer who have had surgery to try to cure their cancer. The researchers hope that by looking for ctDNA in the blood following curative surgery, they can use this information. It might help them to make better decisions on who might need further treatment. And also what the best treatment might be."*[2]

I'll visit a different hospital, the Royal Marsden in Sutton, for my ctDNA tests.

Today marks my first experience at a chemotherapy unit, and I feel a mix of worry and reassurance. I can see how wonderful the doctors and nurses are, which is comforting. However, my enthusiasm dips slightly when it comes to having my blood drawn, especially when the technician walks out with nine bottles for my blood – yes, nine. Fortunately, one of them is just a spare, so they're only taking eight.

I used to be scared of these blood tests, but now they don't bother me as much, although the thought of losing so much blood still concerns me a little.

---

[2] https://www.cancerresearchuk.org/about-cancer/bowel-cancer/treatment/research-clinical-trials/research-diagnosing-treating-bowel-cancer.

As a bonus, I will feel relieved once I find out in eight weeks if I have cancerous DNA. This will help me and my doctors understand a little more about my chances of recurrence and may even guide my treatment plan somewhat.

Another wonderful aspect of today is that I'm getting together with my friends Tommy, Simon and Mark.

Bless them; they come to the village where I live, and we usually meet in the middle. We plan to enjoy a few drinks and a curry together.

It's wonderful to catch up with them. When I began this journal, I was feeling quite unwell during Simon's 50th birthday back in November.

That was the same day I dropped off the FIT test at the doctor's, the very test that ultimately revealed my cancer.

We haven't seen each other since then, and I've obviously been through a lot, but it's truly great to reconnect and discuss what's been happening lately and what I'm about to face. Simon shares a funny story about his colonoscopy that involved him taking both bowel preps at the same time; laughing still hurts me a bit, but it's so great to laugh again.

(And Simon's advice: read the instructions. Don't take both bowel preps on the morning of your colonoscopy. Oooooosh.)

I also learn that my bowel still doesn't appreciate curry. I choose the mildest curry possible, but I'm awakened at one in the morning when that curry decides to make a reappearance.

Oh well, you live and learn, though in my case, I seldom do.

22 February 2025

Today, we have a relaxing day. I feel I should because, frankly, I didn't sleep too well last night since Mr Curry kept trying to make a reappearance.

So, it was nice to chill and unwind. There isn't much to write home about, except that I discovered that having breaded chicken, katsu sauce and white rice seems to go quite well with my stomach.

At least I've found something I can enjoy that isn't too beige, is tasty and doesn't upset my stomach too much.

All in all, this is just a very quiet and relaxing day.

BACK ON THE TREADMILL

23 February 2025

I wake up after 8.5 hours of sleep, and Emma and I go to the gym. Until now, since the operation, all I've done is walk at the gym, but today, I think I'll push myself; it's only 24 hours until it's been six weeks since the op, and I'm going to run. I can't lie; I'm a bit nervous as I start to run, but as I speed up and get comfortable, I feel a surge of delight at finally running again and realising I'm getting ahead in my recovery.

Ultimately, I cover 5.78 km in 29 minutes, and I'm really happy with that.

The thing that spurs me on is that I put on a radio show by a DJ called Ed Mahon, who does a great show called *Cowbell Radio*.[3]

He recently lost his partner in that endeavour to cancer, and as he begins the show, he plays a eulogy to him.

At first, it hits me hard; in the first minute or two, I think about someone dying from cancer.

But then I realise that letting it affect me does no one any good. I'm very sad that it's taken someone else, but if I can overcome it, then hopefully, I can help others.

---

[3] *https://www.edmahonmusic.com/cowbell*.

So, that's what I do. I gradually speed up, running faster and faster. All I want to do is complete the 5 km in 30 minutes. To finish 5.78 in 29 is fantastic.

I feel really good, and I treat Emma and me afterwards to coffee and a pastry from Pret A Manger.

When we return home, Emma and I take the dogs out for a walk, and honestly, I settle in for a day of sports.

I watch my beloved Liverpool beat Man City 2-0 away from home, and some people are singing, "We're going to win the league."

I'd love to sing along with the chant of "Now you're going to believe us," but this whole experience with cancer and this illness teaches me not to count my chickens before they hatch.

Assumptions can make fools of us and even make us feel silly. My goodness, I hope Liverpool wins the league, and I hope this cancer is truly gone. But just like Liverpool, I've got a few more fixtures to overcome before I can say they have won the league and that I've overcome cancer.

24 February 2025

For all intents and purposes, today is just a normal working day. I wake up, walk the dogs, and enjoy it; I'm not hurting as much as I was before. The only pain I have is from my run yesterday, and it's a pain that I welcome. I'm still a bit itchy and sometimes uncomfortable, mainly after eating, but all in all, six weeks post-op, I'm not feeling too bad. So today is about getting settled into work, getting things done and being productive. It's nice to have a day where, apart from this diary, I don't think too much about cancer.

One nice thing that happens is chatting with Suzy, whom I've mentioned in this diary before, and who is the reiki master. Suzy has moved on in her role at work, so we no longer speak daily. I told her I've been writing these diary entries and that she's mentioned in them.

I sometimes wonder whether Suzy knows that I value reiki and will only discover through this diary that I do. We schedule another session for next week, during which we'll have another reiki session. I'll benefit from her expertise, but mainly, I benefit from her friendship because Suzy is a lovely person, and her reiki is magic that I don't understand but truly value.

For those of you undergoing treatment who don't have your very own 'Suzy', it's probably worth noting that both Macmillan and Maggie's offer holistic healing to cancer patients. In a few weeks, I'll be having reiki courtesy of Macmillan. I've included some sources for you below.

- *https://www.macmillan.org.uk/cancer-information-and-support/treatment/coping-with-treatment/complementary-therapies*.
- *https://www.maggies.org/cancer-information/cancer-treatment/types-treatment/complementary-therapies/*.

During the evening, I converse with someone I truly care about – someone I've formed a relationship with over the last few years.

Just so you don't misinterpret this, I mean a platonic relationship, but that doesn't diminish the significance of this person to me. The reason I want to write this entry in my diary is that I hope they might read it, as well as others.

This person trusted me with something incredibly important; the information they shared is something I will never disclose outside of our conversation. However, I include it in my diary because it's vital to talk and share with those you trust. If someone trusts you, in my opinion, you shouldn't try to offer them the 'right' answer. You should strive to provide them with an honest answer based on your experiences, your relationship with them, and empathy, and what you should do is actively listen. Sometimes, people need to let it out; whether it's cancer, physical or mental health, letting somebody speak is so important.

And it's not for me to make light of when somebody shares something with you, but this evening I was watching a programme called *Our Welsh Chapel Dream* with the potter Keith Brymer Jones. This is how he spoke of his relationship, and I believe that this can apply through life.

Keith said that in his relationship, every experience was twice as good, and every problem was half as bad.

I think what he meant by that is that if you surround yourself with the right people, you can double the positives, and if you have the right people, anything negative can feel less severe.

It's through talking to people like this person who trusted me, along with having Emma and many other great people around me, that things haven't been as bad as I initially thought.

If you'd told me a year ago that this was coming, I'm not sure I would've handled it as well as I have. So, this is for you, the reader: if you have someone you care about, listen to them, empathise with them, and perhaps they'll share something that will help them. Similarly, maybe in the future, you can share something with them that benefits both of you. I'm not a wise man, but I'd like to think these thoughts are relatively wise words.

Please show your care for those you love.

25 February 2025

When training for an ultramarathon, the key is consistency. This is something that I'm trying to incorporate into my life in terms of managing cancer.

I still keep referring to it as cancer, even though, technically speaking, it's no longer inside me.

However, there may be rogue cells lingering, which is why I need chemotherapy. I'm viewing the chemotherapy as a 12-week training block. Additionally, I'm working on getting back into good habits after developing poor dietary and exercise habits over the last five weeks.

This morning, I dragged myself out of bed, went to the gym, and completed another 5.7 km in under 30 minutes. My left hamstring is on fire, my right knee hurts, my feet are sore and my chest aches from heavy breathing. Yet, I love every single second of it.

While there, I see Wendy, the receptionist at the colonoscopy unit – the lady I met on 1 December. She advises me to take it easy but also recognises that I'm enjoying myself, which is good for my health.

Outside of this, it's just a normal working day, which I welcome. It feels good to check things off my list. However, I also discover that I need to call the hospital in Guildford because my chemotherapy will begin on 14 March, a Friday. I have to do this to confirm this appointment and one a few days prior.

I'll also need to go into the hospital on 11 March as a new patient, so I must make allowances for that.

This timing disrupts one thing I was hoping for: finishing chemotherapy by my birthday on 24 May.

The likelihood is that, on 24 May, I'll be in the middle of treatment when I feel my worst. But you know what? I'm here for it. If that's how it's got to be, that's how it's got to be. Emma and I may share notes on how shit our birthdays were in 2025, but we'll still be here.

By 1 June, with any luck, in the sixth month of the year, after all of this began in November of last year, I hope to be able to say that I am, for all intents and purposes, cancer-free.

Please keep your fingers crossed for me.

26 February 2025

Today is my last working day of February, a month that has flown by.

Sometimes, I think having a healthy context of time versus reality is beneficial, though as I sit here today, I'm still struggling to know what to eat and I want to eat the right things.

I can't lie; I feel like I've probably overdone it on the exercise front. I'm in a lot of pain in my hip, my groin, my private parts and my stomach wounds; today is my first time taking painkillers for quite a while.

However, I'm just trying to listen to my body, which I've never been very good at. Maybe if I'd paid attention to it earlier, I wouldn't have needed to have a stage three cancerous tumour removed from my body.

I have a good working day, though; I'm so fortunate to have the 'distraction' of work.

During this treatment, everything that used to stress me out no longer does, at least regarding work. I don't see its relative importance, but it has made me a better consultant – possibly more balanced, even calmer and more thoughtful.

This evening, Liverpool beats Newcastle United 2-0. It's a bit of a dress rehearsal for a future cup final. Watching the game, I can't help but think it won't be that easy in March, while also wondering, are we going to win the league?

TURNING AN IDEA INTO A REALITY

27 February 2025

Today is supposed to be a non-working day, but it's quite frantic. The book I co-authored earlier this year is now in demand for International Women's Day events, and my co-author Lucy and I are presenting to people in different companies and organisations throughout this coming week.

Incidentally, and this isn't a plug – but 'events' such as International Women's Day and World Cancer Day have their place. Let's imagine a world of equity and understanding where people are no longer marginalised or treated unfairly. Wouldn't that be lovely!

It's really rewarding to focus on something that's very important to me and doesn't involve the 'C' word.

Additionally, once all of that's done, I have a potential client meeting, which is nice to know, and our friends Michelle and Wayne are coming to visit, so I get to tidy the house – something I haven't been able to do for over six weeks now.

I quite enjoy it, but I do feel a twinge in my left side where one of my scars is. I hope it's just in my mind rather than my body, but it doesn't worry me for now.

Another idea I've been considering is transforming these diary entries into a book.

They currently exist on Substack, but could a printed book and even an audiobook version reach a larger audience? I've contemplated self-publishing, managing everything myself, and donating the profits to charity.

However, I'm also incredibly fortunate to have a publisher: the amazing IT Governance Publishing, a GRC Solutions Company. So today, I reach out to a member of the publishing team who has assisted me with the books I've previously worked on with them.

I ask him if he has a moment for a chat, and he instantly agrees.

We get straight on a Zoom call, and I pitch him the idea of *Shit, I've Got Cancer* being turned into a book or even a series of books. Now, you must understand my publisher doesn't operate in this field. It's normally management and professional-based, but I feel that this topic goes beyond that, and thankfully he agrees. He's unable to promise anything, but he says he'll take it away and come back to me, and maybe, just maybe, *Shit, I've Got Cancer* can be a printed book and an audiobook.

28 February 2025

It's the last day of February, and we get to spend it with Wayne, Michelle, Denise and Tim.

Emma, Michelle, Wayne and I travel 40 minutes to London to meet our friends Denise and Tim. It's a Friday of relaxation.

We have a few drinks, enjoy some lunch and have a really good laugh. It's just a normal day, which, in the context of this diary, probably wouldn't merit an entry.

However, it warrants a significant entry for me because it represents normalcy.

My new normal involves constantly thinking about the tumour that has been removed from me, the chemo that I'm about to undergo, or what I can and cannot eat. Today, I've tried to indulge a bit; I'm not sure if it's good for me, but I do it anyway, and it's incredibly liberating for my mind.

1 March 2025

It's another day of relaxation, though today I can really feel pain in my side from my exercise earlier this week.

I'm not feeling right; I've got pains across all of my scar sites, which also seem to have become a bit scabby again.

Now, the context here is probably nothing majorly wrong, but you can't help but get carried away when you've been in the position I'm in.

I apply abundant thinking, choosing to focus on what I had, not what I feared and end up having a really good day – just another good day of relaxing, eating, mooching around, and having a drink with really good friends, and it's great to have them here.

It's wonderful to be able to have a laugh, to talk about life, to discuss plans, and really just to feel normal again. Thank you, Wayne and Michelle.

2 March 2025

The epitome of a lazy Sunday – we don't do much at all. The four of us go for a walk, grab food, drink, watch TV and football, and just relax.

Wayne and I even manage to have an ice cream since the sun has come out – and can you believe it, we find a 99 (for those outside the UK, it's ice cream in a cone) for £1.00. What a bargain!

The day finishes with a pizza – one I've had a hundred times before, but this time, it wants to tear me apart from the inside out.

As a result, I have an uncomfortable night and feel quite stupid and silly as I keep leaving the room to pass gas.

We laugh about it, but it's quite embarrassing, and my belly won't stop growling after eating this pizza. I know I need to give it time, but it feels like a real step back, which really annoys me.

I just need to get over it, as simple as that.

3 March 2025

Today begins with a public speaking event where Lucy and I are promoting our book, *Allyship Actually*, to a global audience.

What that audience doesn't know is that I've spent most of the night feeling unwell, and my mood is frankly low. I can hide that on the outside, but I can't escape the fact that I'm just not the person I used to be, and it's really, really irritating me.

If I'm honest with myself, I probably drank too much over the weekend. I suspect this is impacting my mood and likely affecting my physical well-being as well. I really just want to be like I used to be – to bounce back, to exercise, to run like I once did, and yes, to enjoy drinking as I once did because I like to enjoy my life. At the moment, I feel like I'm not enjoying my life at all.

As always, this diary is recorded on the day, so I suspect that over the next few days my mood will improve, and I won't feel so down. But today – today is an absolute shitter of a mood.

After work finishes, I have a reiki session with Suzy, and I fall into a Zen-like state. It really is lovely and relaxing. I still have no real idea how it works, but however it works, it's great.

Halfway through the session, I get a phone call from the GP; an appointment had been made earlier today, one which I had declined, but they call anyway.

That appointment is to ask how I'm feeling and to check in on me.

I don't have time to stress about it, and do you know what? Having that chat does wonders for me. It allows me to get things off my chest and express my feelings. I'm pretty sure the reiki and its relaxation helps me manage the conversation.

We're so fortunate to have the NHS. Yes, they may get appointments wrong – but they're still frickin' awesome.

4 March 2025

I'm still in a bad mood. I walk the dogs, but I'm just not feeling it today.

I also have to go to the dentist. This is a pre-chemotherapy dental session, and every single medical appointment I've had over the last six months or so has been crap. I'm completely anticipating this one being crap too.

But it's not. I'm literally in and out in two minutes with a clean bill of health and wished good luck by the dentist for my chemotherapy. This immediately brightens my day, and, on my way out, I say to him, "This is the only positive medical appointment I can recall over these last few months. Thank you."

I return home and begin work, and I'm definitely feeling better as a result of that dental appointment. It's amazing how just a small thing can make you feel better.

In the afternoon, I meet with a nutritionist, a lady named Suzy from Embracing Nutrition, who specialises in cancer care via nutrition. We spend an hour talking, breaking down my diet. Obviously, my diet probably isn't helping me right now, especially the weekend that's just passed. We figure out a way forward for me, though – a way to reintroduce fibre to make me more comfortable and to give me strength in the future with the chemotherapy.

After this meeting, I feel like I'm taking control again, and I think this really helps me, knowing that I'm doing everything I can to get through this.

I also receive an email from an event organiser asking me to attend a ball and sit at the top table as recognition for my work in my industry. I've been feeling on the periphery recently, so to have this in my inbox is really good, but it does present me with a conundrum. I start chemotherapy 14 days before the event, and I've no idea how I'm going to feel. It's also been suggested to me that I should isolate from crowded events because my immune system will be compromised. I really want to go, but I'm not sure it's the right thing to do, and so with the good news comes a tinge of bad because I'm tired of the cancer impacting my day-to-day life in this way.

Well, that said, I definitely feel better than yesterday. I recognise that the alcohol probably made me feel a bit unwell before, so I need to sit down and seriously re-evaluate my priorities right now. Those priorities should definitely start with health and focus on wealth or its absence, as my work is running out. Then, I need to figure out how to enjoy myself amid all of this. When you're dealing with cancer, you're not just dealing with the physical aspect; you're also dealing with not feeling yourself, not being yourself, and even not being able to be yourself. I see these as all distinct issues. You can cover up not feeling yourself, but you can't hide not being yourself. And that's the hardest part because others can see it. That's what worries me.

5 March 2025

There isn't much to report today. I'm still sore, possibly even sorer than I was yesterday. I also have a slight sniffle, almost like a flu-like feeling, but it definitely feels like I pulled a muscle in my lower abdomen.

It stretches down into my groin and is familiar from when I used to run. I use run in the past tense because I think I might have overdone it last week, and that's what I'm suffering from now.

Maybe I need to realise that I'm not the same person I used to be or figure out a way to become the person I used to be. I used to be able to handle overdoing it, but I suspect those days are gone, for now at least.

Tonight, Liverpool go to Paris St Germain, aka PSG. Our goalkeeper is amazing (just like the assistant oncologist), and our defence holds up. We win 1-0 away from home.

Once again, I apologise to people who don't follow football, but for me, this is really important.

It's not about how hard you get hit; it's about how you get up and fight back. That's what Liverpool do tonight, and that's what I'm doing now. I'm also spending over £300 on natural vitamins and minerals, which my nutritionist has told me will be incredibly helpful during chemotherapy. £300!!!

6 March 2025

Today is one of those days when it feels like everything you touch turns to gold, which is wonderful after the last few weeks. I can ease into the day since I'm not working with a client today.

However, Lucy and I later present *Allyship Actually* to a large organisation in the UK. When we join the call, we learn that almost 200 people are joining us, and Lucy and I do a great job, even though we say so ourselves.

We have this presentation down to a T, but more importantly, our messaging is important. This week is International Women's Day and World Book Day, so promoting our book about allyship is a special opportunity.

The audience is fantastic; they listen, learn, ask incredible questions, and provide amazing feedback.

And no sooner have I put the phone down on this call than I receive a message from my publisher asking if I've got a few minutes this afternoon for a chat.

I immediately respond, yes, I'd love to, and we meet up on another Zoom call, where the publisher discusses this book with me.

They would absolutely love to publish *SHIT, I've got Cancer*.

Even better, they share my belief that we could partner with a charity to donate profits from the book to that charity and also help promote the book in the future.

It's such a generous gesture from my publisher. They don't normally work in this area, but ever since I began collaborating with them three or four years ago, they've been incredibly progressive; they've helped me publish books, obviously assisted Lucy, and supported some people we know as well. Right now, what's most special to me is that this diary I'm writing is going to receive a platform that I hope will help others in the future.

I also hope that if and when I fully recover from this disease, that book will continue to exist with or without me, and with or without my cancer, to help others. I believe that's what writing is for, and all of this comes from a kid who barely passed his GCSEs in English.

7 March 2025

Today marks one week away from starting chemotherapy, and a bit like when I had the operation, I'm getting into the mindset of "this time in a week".

I'll understand what I'm facing then. Often, it's the fear of the unknown or the first-time experiences that frighten me. I hope, as with most things in life – and dare I say, including the operation – that in this case, the anticipation will be worse than the reality.

I feel like my pain is improving today, which suggests that I likely harmed myself last week while running. So, I think next time I go to the gym, I'll use a stationary bike and pedal to see if that helps.

Hopefully, it has become clear by now that I'm self-employed. I work as a management consultant in the IT industry. Today was the first day I was informed that I'm a great candidate for an engagement.

However, they said, "We're worried about whether you'll be OK in a stressful environment," and do you know what? I get it. I understand people's concerns for me, and I see why you wouldn't want someone going through chemotherapy putting themselves through the grind to help you out on a job.

Equally, it makes me feel a bit marginalised, not so much for myself, but more for others experiencing what I'm going through, who face similar feedback or are dealing with individuals who aren't honest like those I've encountered. People who say you're not good enough when, in reality, you are. It's just that they don't want to admit they're concerned about hiring someone with cancer or similar socially debilitating illnesses. It's got me thinking about what I want to do for the future.

Maybe there's something I can write or some coaching I can offer to leaders about this subject. To be clear, this is not directed at those who said they weren't sure I could handle it in this particular scenario.

They said to give them a call in a couple of weeks, with no promises attached. "If you're feeling well, we think it could be a good idea" – that's the right way to handle this. I really appreciate how they handle this, but as I mentioned, I worry that not everyone is so honest, and I'd like to try to help people in the future understand what going through cancer and treatment is like.

This will be the last weekend for a couple of weekends when I can actually relax, or at least as far as I know, relax. Because next weekend it's chemotherapy, and the following weekend it's another colonoscopy. I can't lie; I think I've got PTSD when it comes to colonoscopies. Last time I had one, I saw the tumour come on the screen. I really don't want to have to go through that again.

DO NOT SKIP THIS CHAPTER! IMPORTANT INFO WITHIN

This entry is different. It's not about a day; it's about a period – a really important period for anyone dealing with an unexpected illness.

I thought for a long time before adding this chapter. Allowing you into my world is my choice, but in this case, I'm discussing topics that many of us find uncomfortable: money and insurance.

In a world dominated by finances and the belief that "money makes the world go round", this could be the most important chapter you read.

Back in December, my financial advisor (FA) called me. This gentleman is someone I've worked with for approximately 20 years. About 20 years ago, I took out a critical illness and life insurance policy that I've been paying £140 into every month for that entire time.

My FA said, "I think you've got a case here. We should enact your policy." Thus, a process began for making a claim against my critical illness and life insurance policy.

This has been a stressful event. It has been ongoing since December and continues to today, 7 March. As a self-employed individual, I must keep earning.

Despite managing treatment and preparing for chemotherapy, I've persevered with my work. It hasn't been easy, but it hasn't been overly difficult because of my job.

My position allows me to work from home consistently; I'm not climbing ladders, working on a site or driving. I'm at home most days, which has been a blessing for the past three weeks months. I'm also fortunate to have a great client and professional network who have offered me some awesome work over these last few months.

The point of this particular timeout is to say to you, whether you're young, middle-aged, or even old, that if you don't have critical illness and life insurance, please look into it and take it out.

After over three months of proving that I have cancer, it's been difficult. There have been many emails exchanged and phone calls made to prove to my insurer that yes, I do have cancer, that yes, I'm receiving treatment, and that yes, they did operate on me for over five and a half hours to remove a tumour. Fortunately for me, I scanned and filed every letter and test result sent to me by the NHS; please take this onboard as some serious advice!

It's a case of being guilty until proven innocent when it comes to filing a claim, but I understand that insurance companies aren't there to pay out. They exist to take our money, hoping that we don't get ill so they won't have to pay out.

But if you get ill and you have dependents, or even just for yourself, I urge you to consider critical illness and life insurance coverage.

In my case, this week, after three months, we finally settled with the insurance company. The amount of money we received, while it won't make us millionaires overnight or enable us to retire immediately, is enough to provide us with financial stability while I undergo chemotherapy.

This means I have one less stress to worry about regarding finding work and one less stress to worry about when it comes to paying the mortgage. It also means I can focus on writing this book.

The ability to plan for the future is invaluable. Nothing brings reality crashing down like getting ill; for Emma and me, we've realised that we might want to live closer to our friends and support network.

I've realised that I don't want to work to live. While I enjoy work, this whole scenario has altered my perception of its importance. I now harbour a deep desire to write and to help others.

Perhaps, just perhaps, we can achieve that and be nearly mortgage-free by the time we're 50.

This insurance policy has provided us with that flexibility. So, to reiterate, if you have critical illness and life insurance, that's great! But please check the terms to ensure you meet all conditions, as many stipulations exist, and do it now before you need to do so during a high-stress period.

If you don't have a critical illness and life insurance policy, I encourage you to get one.

Do it today!

You may also find yourself in a situation where having financial support is extremely beneficial. I sincerely hope you never encounter such a scenario, but if you do, this advice could be the most crucial part of any book you read.

Please take action now.

Sermon over.

At the back of this book, I will include resources that I hope will be useful to you.

8 March 2025

Today, Emma and I are heading to Brighton to visit some wonderful friends, and it's also International Women's Day.

I mention this because, as a co-author collaborating with Lucy on *Allyship Actually*, we've had a busy week surrounding International Women's Day.

As I've stated in articles elsewhere, this needs to be more than just a week or a day; it must be forever.

Did you know that at the current rate, it will take until the year 2158 for women to achieve equity with men?

Let that sink in: 2158.[4]

This becomes the topic of our conversation when we meet friends in Brighton, along with my cancer, of course.

However, it's good to have conversations that aren't solely focused on that. We engage in debates and have real, intelligent, grown-up discussions. We enjoy a lovely day in Brighton; we walk along the beach and have coffee, and then Emma and I head back home, and I watch Liverpool win 3-1 at home to Southampton.

It's getting closer.

---

[4] *https://www.weforum.org/stories/2024/06/global-gender-gap-2024-what-to-know/*.

After that, we go out for some wine and cheese – a very civilised thing. It's beautiful, and it's nice to start feeling normal finally. Emma and I have a lovely evening; it's good to dress well and feel good again.

I've been struggling with pain recently. I truly believe it's due to overexercising last week, so I've slowed things down.

After speaking with Suzy, the nutritionist, earlier this week, I now have some supplements, and although I'm not sure if they're effective, I feel a lot better.

For that, I'm happy. We're now six days away from beginning chemotherapy. I'm really looking forward to it, not because I want to undergo it, but because I want to finish it. I want this to be over

I want to return to normal, although I'm not sure I'll ever be able to do so.

9 March 2025

I woke up today and thought I drank too much wine last night. I haven't had a glass of wine since before I trained for the ultramarathon over a year ago, but last night, Emma and I went to a new wine bar, which was very civilised, where we ate some cheese and enjoyed some wine.

It was just a nice evening for the two of us to hang out, but this morning, I definitely know I drank wine. Still, having a hangover – though mild – was different from being in pain due to surgery, and it actually felt a bit like a relief.

So today was nice and relaxed. Emma went off to a country house while I stayed home, did some writing, and learned more about chemotherapy and how that will work. I also learned more about how I can adapt my diet to get through chemotherapy.

I also sat down and went through our finances. We've been thinking about moving out of our current home to somewhere where we have less of a mortgage to pay.

Recent events have meant that we're re-evaluating our priorities in life and wondering if we could move somewhere closer to friends where we'd have more support.

It's a sad fact that I'm now more likely to have a cancer recurrence than I was to get cancer in the first place. As much as I don't think it'll come, I've always been prepared for the worst and hoping for the best.

So, we started thinking about where we could move to in order to get support, save money, and rationalise our mortgages. Maybe it's a pipe dream, or perhaps it's a new idea to consider as we adapt to our new normal. However, I actually quite enjoy doing the maths. I enjoy doing the research, and this evening, Emma's parents came over. We had a bite to eat and talked about what opportunities might be available.

We also received amazing news. You may recall that Emma's father, Terry, has been battling cancer. He has prostate cancer – or should I say, HAD.

He underwent radiotherapy treatment in January and February, and today he found out that he's received the all-clear. This is great news.

One down, one to go.

10 March 2025

Today, I realise that these diary entries are now almost four months old. Writing something every day hasn't been too challenging, but today has been the first day I feel like there's not much to report; it's been so quiet.

I try to write this diary in the evening, but sometimes, I'll start in the morning on my dog walk, revisiting it in the afternoon and evening.

Today, it's quiet, but then something happens, and there's loads to report.

It's just a normal day. I'm quietly going about my business working and just thinking about my next steps.

You see, I've got five days left from my current client; I've been working with them month to month since November, thankfully they needed me beyond January when I thought that might be our last time working together. It's a situation we're all comfortable with, and I thank them for their support.

It's at this point that I now need to figure out if I'm going to continue working with them, what that will look like and whether they accept the statement of work I put together; second to that, they need to see if they have the finances in place to continue our work together.

And, of course, with chemotherapy on the horizon, both parties need to ensure that we can accommodate my illness in the context of the work that must be delivered.

Earlier in the diary, I included a longer piece on life and critical illness cover.

Today, that importance strikes home when my insurer contacts me and informs me that Emma and I will be receiving a payment. While it's not absolutely life-changing, it'll help us during my chemotherapy. It means I don't have to worry about work and can relax if needed.

To reiterate, look into insurance; it could be really useful for you in the future.

I don't know whether it's this good news or the supplements I've been taking recently, but I'm beginning to feel a bit more human, which is ironic really as I'll be starting chemotherapy on Friday, and I've no idea whether I'll feel human or not while doing that, but it's three months, so I figure, why not just live with it and crack on.

Later in the day, I reach out to Bowel Cancer UK to ask if they'd be interested in partnering. It's really good for me because I've recently joined a committee focused on cancer research, and I'm now going to dedicate my voluntary time to that. I'm hoping we can build a partnership that spreads these diary entries and the messages within them to a larger audience and, hopefully, help someone in their moment of need in the future.

11 March 2025

Today could be considered 'one of those days'; I suppose you might call it a day of two halves. The first half was simple. We got up, had coffee, walked the dogs, and worked in the morning.

Nice and easy.

In the afternoon, we drove to Guildford, which is about 45 minutes away, for an appointment at St Luke's, the Cancer Hospital. This is where I'll be having my chemotherapy.

Honestly, I wasn't sure what this appointment was about. I noticed it was a group appointment, which instantly made me feel uneasy; sitting in a group is not something I particularly enjoy.

In the letter we received for the appointment, we were asked to watch a video – in fact, three videos – all of which I made sure to view. If someone gives me homework, I do it!

One video covered chemotherapy, the other discussed having a PICC line installed, and another focused on the drugs I'll be taking.

Each video discussed the side effects of our poor health, and they all annoyed me by suggesting that the solution was to eat cakes, biscuits and more chocolate to counteract any side effects.

Now, I know they don't mean it literally, but come on, I don't want to end up at the end of this treatment with diabetes, as well as – I hope – being a cancer survivor.

When we entered the room, there were 12 of us: 6 patients and 6 loyal family members or friends. The first thing we were asked was whether we had watched the videos. The majority answered yes, but then we were told, "We have to show you the videos anyway."

Why ask us to watch them if we have to see them again?

I know it's not a big deal, but I had to take half a day off work – a day during which I'm not earning money – to sit in a room and watch 45 minutes of videos again that I never wanted to see in the first place.

We were then spoken to by a lovely lady who works in the alternative therapist element of the hospital. Followed by a dietician who recommended more cake, more chocolate, and more biscuits, and our lovely nurse who took us all through the treatments and told us all the side effects once more.

Emma and I had also been having some debate as to whether my treatment would be a full four-week form of one intravenous treatment and four weeks of tablets or three weeks formed of one intravenous treatment plus three weeks of tablets and a week off.

Indeed, this is how it'll function. I will attend the hospital every three weeks. I'll have my intravenous treatment for two to three hours and then go home. Once I'm home, I'll take another chemotherapy drug for two weeks and then have a week's break. In that interim week, I'll have a blood test to see if I'm ready for the next round of treatment.

At the end of the session, I asked the nurse how many treatments I'd be having. She suggested it would be six, which may go down to four.

If it's six, this will take me through to the end of June, and I don't want to go through this until the end of June. It'll be, give or take, seven to eight months of dealing with this cancer.

I'll need to have a phone consultation with my chemotherapy specialist on the Wednesday before every treatment, and once a week, I'll need to see a district nurse to get my PICC line dressed.

I'm going to sound ungrateful here, but I've always recorded these diary entries in the moment, and it's how I feel.

I'm sitting here tonight about to watch Liverpool play Paris St Germain, and frankly, I'm pissed off.

I feel like I was led to believe this would be a straightforward three months, but the truth is I probably only heard three months and ran with it. So, as I record this diary entry, I'm bringing myself down from the ceiling and realising that maybe next time I should listen better. Even in this case, having two of us there didn't result in us having the correct information; in fact, we got it wildly wrong.

So, if you're following my path, my advice to you is two things.

First, don't watch the videos before arriving; you'll have to watch them again. You may as well lose 45 minutes of your life instead of 90.

Second, during your first meeting with the oncologist, bring a pen and paper, and ask, "How many treatments will I be having?"

Third, ask how long your treatment will last.

If you do this, then you, unlike me, will not drive home and say to your wife, "Stop the diet. I'm going to the chippy to buy chips, scampi and mushy peas," when all I really want is 12 pints to fall into oblivion.

And by the way, I just had the chips, scampi and mushy peas, and to rub chip salt in the wound, our local chippy only takes cash. I thought I had the exact amount of money, but it turned out that three of my pound coins were euros, so I now owe the guy in the chippy £3.

I left the shop with my tail between my legs, feeling completely embarrassed.

I'm now recording this before Liverpool plays Paris Saint Germain in the Champions League, so let's see what mood I'm in tomorrow based on the score.

12 March 2025

Well, Liverpool lost last night. That dampens the mood after losing on penalties as well. Oh well, you can't win them all.

Poor Emma is unwell. She's got a cough that's keeping us both up at night, and now, of course, we're both worried that I'll get that cough just in time for my chemotherapy in two days.

It's amazing how I don't want chemotherapy; however, I also don't want a cold to prevent me from starting the treatment. I just want to get this ball rolling because the sooner it starts, the sooner it can be stopped.

As I've still got pain in my lower abdomen, I spoke to the MacMillan nurses earlier, who are fantastic. I don't think it's anything to worry about. I'm pretty sure I overdid it a couple of weeks ago, but I've been ramping up my walking with the dogs, and that's helping, and a bit of stretching seems to help.

It's with that in mind that I speak to Macmillan about my joining some yoga classes, and so starting on 21 of March, I'm going to be doing yoga and trying to get rid of this little pain in my stomach that's holding me back. I might even go there and take advantage of the counselling services because I'm still bricking it about my upcoming colonoscopy.

I can't seem to shake the fear or the PTSD of having seen my tumour the last time I was on one of those beds.

My advice to you, the reader, is if you're going for a colonoscopy, firstly, it's very unlikely to be the worst-case scenario. I'm just one of the unlucky ones.

Secondly, you might want to close your eyes, as seeing your insides isn't the nicest thing. If there's anything up there, removing the image from your head is impossible, at least in my case.

Today's good thing was speaking with the Bowel Cancer UK research team. They're keen to take this diary and partner with my publisher as we turn this into a book.

My thinking is as follows: this could be a series of books broadly broken up into:

- **Number one:** diagnosis and surgery. Hopefully, this is the book you're reading now.
- **Number two:** recovery and chemotherapy.
- **Number three:** chemotherapy all clear/next steps/recovery and an attempt to move on.

I'm sitting here on 12 March writing this, and I'm not sure if it'll come true, but I would like to release this book as a series. I'd like to include a challenge that I'm setting for myself to finally run a half-marathon and a marathon to benefit one or two charities.

13 March 2025

Last night, I slept in the spare room. My wife Emma has a cold, and we're both worried that I might catch it. She's quite unwell, so I spend a lot of today gathering bits and bobs to make sure she's catered for.

In the morning, I walk the dogs and decide to go to the gym, where I sit on a cycling machine for 30 minutes. This is the first time I've ever done this, and it's quite boring. However, I'm still unsure if I can run right now, as I still have a bit of pain in my stomach. That said, it does feel like somebody has dialled down that pain overnight, and I wonder if it's related to my having a great night's sleep last night.

I'm not technically working today, but I have a meeting with my publisher to discuss turning these diary entries into a book. In another turn of events, I meet with a publisher in the United States to discuss an altogether different book.

Both are quite exciting, and I'm wondering if I'm slowly becoming a full-time writer rather than an IT consultant.

As the day wears on, Emma isn't well. She also has a lower immune system due to some drugs that she has to take for an autoimmune disease, so we need to keep an eye on her. We also need her to come with me tomorrow to the first chemotherapy treatment, and we're not quite sure what to do.

Also as the day wears on, I start to get a bit of a sore throat, but I'm pretty sure it's just because Emma is unwell, and it's not a real sore throat.

I take my temperature, and I'm at 37°, so that seems fine. Here we are on Chemotherapy Eve, and I'm about to finish a fantastic series that I started, or should I say restarted in terms of season one during my surgery?

The Wire.

If you haven't seen the HBO series *The Wire*, I thoroughly recommend it. It really is well-paced, but it's one of those shows that doesn't care if you're looking at your phone; it's going to give you about 50 details that you might miss. So, it really rewards you as you watch it and as you go through the seasons. I had planned on finishing it during chemo tomorrow, but I started five episodes today, and I can't put it down. It's really, really good.

So, I guess this is the end of my surgery and recovery phase, and with any luck and no cold, tomorrow begins my chemotherapy phase.

WHAT NEXT?

Thank you for taking this journey with me! Your support and willingness to share in these experiences mean the world. Remember, life can throw us curveballs, but we are not alone!

Unlike most books, I, as the author, cannot tell you the ending because I have no idea what it is myself.

With any luck, I start chemotherapy tomorrow and cruise through it, although if you were to look online or see the testimonies of others, it might seem unlikely that I simply sail through.

Keeping this diary has effectively kept me sane, and being able to give something back to you, the reader, in the hopes that it helps you is my motivation.

For my physical and mental health, I know I need to get through this next 12 to 16 weeks of chemotherapy. As I mentioned, I must treat this as if I am a boxer or someone training for a marathon.

I need to focus on my end goal, which I hope is to go into remission and remove any cancerous cells from my body. I cannot lie; I sit here today, the day before my chemotherapy, still in pain from my operation, although it's nowhere near as bad as it was previously.

Mentally, I am scarred; I still cannot shake the feeling that maybe one day, this cancer will come and take me away from the world.

What next?

This is a negative spin on the situation, but I do not always feel that way; this is thanks to the support of Emma, my family, my friends, and every colleague who has supported me throughout this journey.

I also want to acknowledge the NHS and every cancer specialist who has helped, not to mention the support I have received from readers in whatever form they have encouraged me.

I feel like I will get through this, which is why this book does not end with:

"The End." It concludes with, "What next?"

After reading this book, I hope you find something within it that helps you or enables you to assist someone close to you. I sincerely hope you will return to join me on this journey through chemotherapy recovery and what I hope will be a new life post-cancer. Moreover, I will not forget this experience and will do everything I can to help others.

I am already preparing for Part 2 of this journey.

This next set of diary entries will dive into the world of chemotherapy – a topic that can understandably evoke feelings of fear; I certainly feel that way.

However, I believe that humour has an undeniable power in helping us cope with reality. I just hope I can laugh more than cry during this next phase.

If you would like to reach out, please see my email address below:

david@solsevenstudio.com

What next?

With love, and a massive fuck you to cancer.

BOWEL CANCER UK REFERENCES

Below are some references that I have found to be super useful in my treatment.

Bowel Cancer UK: Not only as supporters of this book but with an easy-to-navigate website offering information and a forum to speak with others who are undergoing a similar journey.

Below are useful pages to include, but are not limited to:

- Bowel Cancer UK home page: *https://www.bowelcanceruk.org.uk/*.
- Bowel Cancer UK news page: *https://www.bowelcanceruk.org.uk/news-and-blogs/news/*.
- Bowel Cancer UK community page: *https://community.bowelcanceruk.org.uk/*.
- Bowel Cancer UK – Ask the Nurse: *https://www.bowelcanceruk.org.uk/how-we-can-help/ask-the-nurse/*.

Bowel Cancer UK – publications, booklets and factsheets. This page also contains questions to ask medical professionals: *https://www.bowelcanceruk.org.uk/about-bowel-cancer/our-publications/*.

After the surgery: *https://www.bowelcanceruk.org.uk/about-bowel-cancer/treatment/surgery/after-surgery/*.

Other Cancer support charities

- Macmillan Cancer Support: *https://www.macmillan.org.uk/*.
- Maggie's: *https://www.maggies.org/*.
- Cancer Research UK: *https://www.cancerresearchuk.org/*.
- Cancer Support UK: *https://cancersupportuk.org/*.

Mental Health and Well-being

Each charity listed above can provide mental health and well-being services; I include some more here for your reference.

- Samaritans: *https://www.samaritans.org/*.
- Shout: *https://giveusashout.org/*.
- Mind: *https://www.mind.org.uk/*.
- ANDYSMANCLUB: *https://andysmanclub.co.uk/*.
- NHS UK: *https://www.nhs.uk/nhs-services/mental-health-services/*.

Critical illness and Life Insurance References

Due to my geographical location, I have focused on the UK market. If you are an international reader, please take the time to research critical illness and life insurance coverage in your region or country.

- "Types of insurance", Citizens Advice: *https://www.citizensadvice.org.uk/consumer/insurance/types-of-insurance/*.
- "10 Tips To Help You Choose The Right UK Health Insurance", The Private Healthcare Company:

https://www.the-phc.co.uk/10-tips-to-choose-the-right-uk-health-insurance.

- "Best private health insurance 2025", Which?: *https://www.which.co.uk/money/insurance/health-insurance/get-the-best-private-health-insurance-a2BPc9a7R62E.*
- "Best critical illness cover UK: Who offers the best critical illness cover in 2025?", Reassured: *https://www.reassured.co.uk/critical-illness/best-critical-illness-cover-uk/.*
- Top 10 best private health insurance companies UK (2025), myTribe *https://www.mytribeinsurance.co.uk/knowledge/best-private-health-insurance-uk.*
- What Is The UK's Best Critical Illness Insurance in 2025?", Drewberry™: *https://www.drewberryinsurance.co.uk/critical-illness-insurance/guides/what-is-the-best-critical-illness-cover.*
- "Top 26 Critical Illness Life Insurance Policies", Our Life Plan: *https://ourlifeplan.co.uk/critical-illness-insurance/.*
- "2025 UK Life Insurance Statistics", Forbes: *https://www.forbes.com/uk/advisor/life-insurance/life-insurance-statistics/.*
- "Unlocking the Future of the Critical Illness Insurance Market: Growth Rate, Key Trends, and Opportunities for 2025-2034", The Business Research Company:

Bowel Cancer UK references

https://blog.tbrc.info/2025/03/critical-illness-insurance-market-trends-2/.

FURTHER READING

GRC Solutions is the world's leading publisher for governance and compliance. Our industry-leading pocket guides, books and training resources are written by real-world practitioners and thought leaders. They are used globally by audiences of all levels, from students to C-suite executives.

Our high-quality publications cover all IT governance, risk and compliance frameworks and are available in a range of formats. This ensures our customers can access the information they need in the way they need it.

Other books you may find useful include:

- *Allyship Actually – Why it's 'We' and not 'Me'* by Lucy Grimwade and David Barrow, *www.itgovernance.co.uk/shop/product/allyship-actually-why-its-we-and-not-me*

- *An Education in Service Management – A guide to building a successful service management career and delivering organisational success* by David Barrow, *www.itgovernance.co.uk/shop/product/an-education-in-service-management-a-guide-to-building-a-successful-service-management-career-and-delivering-organisational-success*

- *Well-being in the Workplace – A guide to resilience for individuals and teams* by Sarah Cook, *www.itgovernance.co.uk/shop/product/well-being-in-the-workplace-a-guide-to-resilience-for-individuals-and-teams*

For more information on GRC Solutions and IT Governance™, a GRC Solutions Company as well as branded publishing services, please visit *https://www.itgovernance.co.uk/*.

Branded publishing

Through our branded publishing service, you can customise our publications with your organisation's branding. For more information, please contact:

clientservices-uk@grcsolutions.io

Related services

GRC Solutions offers a comprehensive range of complementary products and services to help organisations meet their objectives.

For a full range of resources, please visit *www.itgovernance.co.uk*.

Training services

GRC Solutions' training programme is built on our extensive practical experience designing and implementing management systems based on ISO standards, best practice and regulations.

Our courses help attendees develop practical skills and comply with contractual and regulatory requirements. They also support career development via recognised qualifications.

Learn more about our training courses and view the full course catalogue at

www.itgovernance.co.uk/training.

Professional services and consultancy

We are a leading global consultancy of IT governance, risk management and compliance solutions. We advise organisations around the world on their most critical issues and present cost-saving and risk-reducing solutions based on international best practice and frameworks.

We offer a wide range of delivery methods to suit all budgets, timescales and preferred project approaches.

Find out how our consultancy services can help your organisation at

www.itgovernance.co.uk/consulting.

Industry news

Want to stay up to date with the latest developments and resources in the IT governance and compliance market? Subscribe to our Security Spotlight newsletter and we will send you mobile-friendly emails with fresh news and features about your preferred areas of interest, as well as unmissable offers and free resources to help you successfully start your project: *www.itgovernance.co.uk/security-spotlight-newsletter.*

EU for product safety is Stephen Evans, The Mill Enterprise Hub, Stagreenan, Drogheda, Co. Louth, A92 CD3D, Ireland. (servicecentre@itgovernance.eu)

www.ingramcontent.com/pod-product-compliance
Lightning Source LLC
Chambersburg PA
CBHW050805270326
41926CB00025B/4540